THE HEALTHCARE EXECUTIVE'S GUIDE TO URGENT CARE CENTERS AND FREESTANDING EDs

MICHAEL F. BOYLE, MD, FACEP

DANIEL G. KIRKPATRICK, MHA, FACHE

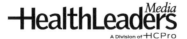

HealthLeaders *Media*

A Division of HCPro

+HCPro

The Healthcare Executive's Guide to Urgent Care Centers and Freestanding EDs is published by HealthLeaders Media

Copyright © 2012 HealthLeaders Media

All rights reserved. Printed in the United States of America.   5   4   3   2   1

ISBN: 978-1-60146-933-5

HCPro, Inc., provides information resources for the healthcare industry.

HCPro, Inc., is not affiliated in any way with The Joint Commission, which owns the JCAHO and Joint Commission trademarks.

Michael F. Boyle, MD, FACEP, Author

Daniel G. Kirkpatrick, MHA, FACHE, Author

Carrie Vaughan, Editor

Bob Wertz, Managing Editor

Matt Cann, Group Publisher

Doug Ponte, Cover Designer

Mike Mirabello, Senior Graphic Artist

Matt Sharpe, Production Manager

Shane Katz, Art Director

Jean St. Pierre, Senior Director of Operations

Advice given is general. Readers should consult professional counsel for specific legal, ethical, or clinical questions. Arrangements can be made for quantity discounts. For more information, contact:

HCPro, Inc.

75 Sylvan Street, Suite A-101

Danvers, MA 01923

Telephone: 800-650-6787 or 781-639-1872

Fax: 800-639-8511

Email: *customerservice@hcpro.com*

HCPro, Inc., is the parent company of HealthLeaders Media.

Visit HealthLeaders Media online at *www.healthleadersmedia.com*

Rev. 10/2012
51757

Contents

Contents

Contents

About the Authors

Michael F. Boyle, MD, FACEP

Michael F. Boyle, MD, FACEP, has spent more than 20 years practicing emergency medicine and managing emergency departments, fast track programs, occupational medicine programs, and urgent care centers. He is the regional medical director at Traverse City, Michigan–based Emergency Consultants, Inc., managing sites in New York, Delaware, and Pennsylvania.

Dr. Boyle has traveled extensively providing consultation for emergency department management, hospital wide flow improvement, and patient satisfaction. His main focus is hospital-affiliated programs for emergency services, occupational medicine, and urgent care. Dr. Boyle currently oversees three urgent care sites, and he will soon be opening an additional urgent care and free standing emergency department. Dr. Boyle received his degree from Eastern Virginia Medical School in Norfolk, Virginia, and completed his emergency medicine residency at Wright State University of Medicine in Dayton, Ohio.

Daniel G. Kirkpatrick, MHA, FACHE

Daniel G. Kirkpatrick, MHA, FACHE, has more than 30 years of healthcare management experience in consulting, staff, and administrator roles. He leads client services at BestPractices, Inc., an emergency medicine leadership and staffing practice affiliate of EmCare. Mr. Kirkpatrick has extensive consulting experience working with group practices and hospitals in meeting operational/financial goals, as well as enhancing service, leadership, safety, and sustainability performance.

Prior work experience in public accounting, administrative roles in hospitals (for-profit, nonprofit, specialty medical-surgical, and behavioral health), and extensive practice management for medical practices (primary care, specialty, and hospital-based) provide him sensitivity to the complex issues confronting healthcare providers. Dan holds a BA in Psychology from the College of Wooster and an MHA from The Ohio State University.

Dan, his wife, and children live in eastern North Carolina.

Acknowledgments

Many people have assisted in the production of this book and to all of you I am truly grateful. I would like to specifically acknowledge Dr. Robert Williams, chairman of the board at Emergency Consultants Inc., who has always served as a mentor and provided extensive education and advice on healthcare economics and the political environment. Several colleagues provided specific information on staffing, program expansion, and other topics. I would like to thank Dr. Jospura and Dr. Richard Koehler, who serves as medical director for our urgent care sites, and Dr. Richard Conyers for his occupational medicine expertise. Several of our site nurse managers provided information on staffing, supplies, and clinic start up including Ms. Lori Greeney from Oswego Health and Ms. Kristina Gambitta and Ms. Amy Thomas, who are both from our programs with Cayuga Medical Center. In addition, I would like to thank John Fraley and Tammy Antoncic from SymMetrix Revenue Solutions for their assistance with billing and coding information. I would also like to thank Dan, my coauthor, for making this book possible, and for the trips across the country providing facilities with our expertise.

Finally, I am thankful for all of the blessings bestowed upon me and the love of my life, Bobbi (my wife), who has stood by me for more than 20 years, and my daughters, Marcianna and Victoria, who have tolerated my many hours of work away from home. Thank you and I love you all.

—*Michael F. Boyle, MD, FACEP*

Acknowledgments

I've had the privilege of befriending and working with Mike Boyle over the past six years, and a truer colleague doesn't exist! Having this opportunity to collaborate on a work that "teases out" some of the nuances of this burgeoning field of urgent care medicine has been wonderful.

Special thanks to Jaime Vance, Mike Drinkwater, and the staff of Martin Gottlieb and Associates for assisting with coding and billing, explaining the inherent complexities, and their willingness to participate in advancing this body of knowledge.

I'm indebted to Drs. Kirk Jensen and Thom Mayer who have both whetted my appetite for emergency medicine service delivery and challenged me to never forget that the patient always comes first.

The steadfast support, understanding, and patience of a loving wife cannot be overstated. This project was of particular interest because she offered her nursing perspective which was very helpful—thanks, Allison. Home base for me is my family and special thanks to my kids, of whom I am very proud: Dave and Dawn; Steven and Lindsay; Travis; Stephen; and Austin.

A special thanks to my partners in Four Guys, a healthcare consulting venture—everyone needs differing perspectives to stay grounded and honest—and Dave, Tony, and Jim fill that bill very well!

—Daniel G. Kirkpatrick, MHA, FACHE

Introduction

The intent of this book is to provide both the healthcare executive and entrepreneurial physician basic tools to research and consider implementing an urgent care center. The following are the major aspects of urgent care centers covered in this book:

- The major political changes leading to the development and rapid increase of urgent care centers and freestanding emergency departments (ED) in the past five years

- The certificate of need and other statutes for the corporate practice of medicine regarding urgent care centers

- The different types of urgent care, including retail clinics, cash clinics, moderate- and high-level urgent care, and freestanding EDs, along with indications for the development of each

- The five basic reasons for a healthcare system to expand into the urgent care market

- A step-by-step analysis of the urgent care business plan development process, urgent care site selection, and proforma development

- The various staffing levels required based on the intent of the urgent care site including medical technicians, licensed vocational nurses, registered nurses, nurse practitioners, and physicians

- The basic marketing plans and patient satisfaction methods to promote growth and volume for the site

- The benefits of developing a full-service occupational medicine program

- The methods for urgent care center expansion, such as the performance of physical examinations, travel medicine, and immunization clinics

- The unique challenges faced by freestanding EDs

We hope that this information provides adequate guidance for administrators in the basic understanding of urgent care programs. In addition, we strive to provide the physician with necessary information for the development of an urgent care site in the hope that appropriate planning leads to future success of the clinic.

Healthcare Market for Urgent Care Centers and Freestanding EDs

Healthcare costs continue to escalate in both the public and private sectors. Reasons for this include the increased cost and availability of advanced technology (e.g., MRI, CT), poorly controlled costs with end-of-life care, overtesting by providers due to fear of litigation, overtesting at the demand of the patient (e.g., MRI tests for back pain), fraud and abuse of Medicare/Medicaid, excessive charges for prescription drugs, and cost shifting by hospitals to cover uninsured and/or indigent care, among others.

The economic downturn in 2008, starting with the collapse of the mortgage industry, has resulted in further pressures on the U.S. healthcare system. For example, the unemployment rate was more than 9% in 2011,[1] which lead to people losing healthcare coverage, delaying elective surgeries, and forgoing treatment. The current economic climate has still not yielded answers or improvement to rising healthcare costs. U.S. companies continue to decrease reimbursement for healthcare coverage by increasing cost sharing (increased copays) with employees or eliminating coverage altogether.[2]

As a result of these market pressures, the number of people without insurance has escalated and will likely exceed 50 million in 2012.[3] This number does not include people who are underinsured. A significant number of the uninsured population is probably unable to afford the average $1,500 per month cost of insurance. There is, however, a select population of young and healthy employed individuals who elect not to purchase health insurance and play healthcare roulette by avoiding the premium expense.

Changing Insurance Landscape

As health insurance has gone from covering only catastrophic healthcare events, which are a large cause of financial ruin and bankruptcy in the United States, to routine care, the general public has the expectation that there will be very little out-of-pocket expense. But now, the pendulum is rapidly shifting to greater costs forced onto the consumer and away from the employer as companies eliminate coverage or increase the portion employees pay.

The original intent of insurance was the development of financial risk shifting from the patient to the insurance carrier.[4] Due to the economic conditions after World War II, wage increases were frozen by the government, forcing employers to look for alternative incentives to improve a financial package for prospective employees. This was the beginning of the provision of healthcare and other benefits as a means to supplement income, also known as the "fringe benefit error." Employer-sponsored health benefits were untaxed income to the employee. But during the past few decades, insurance benefits have grown from simple catastrophic care to include routine physical exams, health screenings, prescription drugs, and hospitalization. These added benefits come with a cost to the purchaser of the policy: the employer.

The cost of healthcare became too high for many employers to continue to foot the bill, in part because, with limited out-of pocket costs, consumers often utilize greater healthcare services. The classic example of this trend is end-of-year medical care. After consumers have used up their annual health insurance deductible, they will try to schedule an elective surgery or colonoscopy screening because of the decrease in the out-of-pocket costs they are responsible for once their deductible has been met. If the procedure or test will not cost the consumer money, utilization will likely be higher.

Between 2000 and 2009, employer-sponsored private health insurance declined from 67% to 58%.[5] As a result, patients became more responsible for their personal healthcare costs through increased copays, provision of their own insurance, or paying out of pocket for healthcare services. It is likely that patients will be more discriminating in expenditures when cost of care comes out of pocket versus from an insurance company or government source. Part of the discrimination will include both cost and quality—especially as this type of information becomes more easily accessible and just a keystroke away on the Internet through the Hospital Compare and Hospital Consumer Assessment of Healthcare Provider and Systems websites. Patients are also becoming better-educated consumers of healthcare.

Major purchasers of healthcare will begin to steer patients to more cost-effective alternatives to receive care, such as urgent care centers versus hospital emergency departments (ED). One major change is the source of healthcare funding. In our experience as a large provider of emergency and urgent care services, 2011 was the first year that Medicare and Medicaid accounted for greater than 50% of all billed patients, which means that the bulk of healthcare is financed by state and federal resources. The majority of healthcare costs involves hospital care, physician/provider fees, and prescription drugs.

Costs of Care

Much of our discussion reviews costs of care and patient charges. In this context, we use cost to identify how much it costs healthcare facilities to provide the care. From the patient aspect, we identify charges as the fee paid by the patient.

In some cases, the cost of caring for a patient in urgent care clinics may be lower and the charge to the patient for this care may also be lower in urgent care clinics. The reason for these differences in cost is most often related to the lower overhead of these types of facilities (e.g., size of the facility and the cost of staffing). Retail clinics, for example, often have minimal space and are staffed by a single nurse practitioner resulting in both minimal costs and minimal charges.

As urgent care clinics grow in complexity, from offering basic to advanced services, the clinic must pay for additional office space and staffing requirements, such as clerical personnel, that result in both cost and charge increases. Obviously, staffing urgent care centers with physicians versus nurse practitioners or physician assistants is a more expensive alternative but would be required to deliver higher levels of care.

When the urgent care center is affiliated with a hospital, it will often see and treat all patients (including Medicaid and self-pay) without collecting fees prior to delivery of services resulting in bad debt and cost shifting, whereas privately owned facilities sometimes do not accept Medicaid or self-pay patients unless cash is paid up front.

As we discuss later in Chapter 6, a major cost advantage of urgent care clinics over EDs is the lack of overnight coverage. EDs must have the staff available 24 hours per day, 7 days per week, which can be expensive when volumes are typically lower from the hours of 2 a.m. until 7 a.m. Urgent care clinics are usually open during peak flow hours and benefit during the entire time of operations, which maximizes productivity and minimizes costs.

A key point for both healthcare executives and governmental officials to understand, however, is the vital need for full-service, hospital-based EDs and the unique reasons for differences in both facility cost and patient charges. The number of EDs in the United States continues to decline in the approximately 4,700 hospital-based facilities nationwide. According to *USA Today*, closures of nonrural EDs exceeded 27%, with a drop from 2,446 to 1,779 from 1990 through 2009.[6] Yet, our nation's EDs represent only 3% of the national healthcare expenditure, which exceeds $2 trillion dollars.[7] The general population, media, and politicians believe that EDs are expensive places to receive care, but when you understand the fundamental staffing costs of an ED visit at 2 a.m., the marginal cost for an emergency visit is actually very low.[8]

On the other hand, the cost to keep an urgent care clinic open past 11 p.m. may be too high to remain viable, suggesting that EDs are still the most viable option in the late evening and early morning hours for some nonemergent cases. According to Robert Williams, MD, the marginal costs of care for minor patient injuries are low in the ED.[9] We firmly believe that both costs and charges for nonemergent cases can be reduced in urgent care clinics but argue that urgent care centers that stay open 24 hours per day lose a significant component of costs savings and result in charge increases.

Access to Care

One of the key challenges the U.S. healthcare industry grapples with is access to care. There are roughly 50 million Americans who lack healthcare insurance.[10] Healthcare reform addresses this need and offers funding paying for services. According to the Congressional Budget Office, more than 30 million Americans will have access to healthcare coverage when healthcare reform under The Patient Protection and Affordable Care Act (PPACA) takes effect.[11]

Yet, providing healthcare coverage to more Americans does not ensure healthcare access. Coverage also must provide competitive reimbursement to have physician practices open their doors to these patients, as we learned from Massachusetts healthcare reform. In 2006, the state of Massachusetts mandated universal healthcare coverage. The law stated that residents of Massachusetts obtain a state government-regulated minimum level of healthcare insurance coverage. It provides free healthcare insurance for residents earning less than 150% of the federal poverty level (FPL) who are not eligible for Mass Health and also partially subsidizes healthcare insurance for those earning up to 300% of the FPL.[12]

The state covered more than 430,000 patients, combining individual mandates, insurance reforms, and publically subsidized insurance product starting in 2006.[13] The majority of these patients were covered through the state's Medicaid program that eliminated costs as a factor for avoidance of healthcare that has been suggested by many.[14] Massachusetts boasts one of the highest primary care physician–to–population ratio compared to many states, but many residents continue to have difficulty with access to care.[15] ED utilization continued to increase despite healthcare reform, and access to care continued to be problematic for the newly insured population.[16] Primary care physicians with closed patient panels may be a significant reason for access issues despite the increased per-capita availability of physicians in Massachusetts.[17]

Roughly 60 million Americans, or nearly one in five, lack adequate access to primary care due to a shortage of primary care physicians in their communities.[18] In many areas, access to primary care is challenging even for patients who have an established relationship with a physician. Same-day or next-day appointments are still difficult for these patients to obtain.[19] People without insurance have little to no access to a primary care office outside of urgent care centers and EDs for minor medical conditions. Evaluation for minor illness and injuries are often referred to the ED rather than being seen in the private office, and fewer physicians accept patients with Medicaid due to poor levels of reimbursement.[20]

Physician access is further impaired by shortages of primary care providers across the United States, with a projected deficit of more than 60,000 physicians by 2015.[21] According to the Association of American Medical Colleges, up to one-third of the physician population will retire in the next decade.[22]

One solution to access includes a change in the continuum of care. Many primary care physicians will become responsible for health maintenance, routine care of common medical conditions (e.g., asthma/chronic obstructive pulmonary disorder [COPD], diabetes, hypertension, etc.), with little time to focus on acute illnesses. Urgent care centers fill in this niche to deliver unscheduled healthcare services for illness and injuries. Expansion of hours beyond normal physician office hours and offering weekend and holiday access makes urgent care centers a vital component in the healthcare system that can help answer the need for increased patient access to healthcare.

Urgent care centers can also reduce costs of care, alleviate the strain of over-stretched hospital EDs, and become profit centers when planned and managed appropriately. According to the Urgent Care Association of America (UCAOA), there are more than 8,700 urgent care centers in the United States, with projected growth of 300 additional centers per year. Most of these sites are owned by physicians or physician groups, with less than 30% being under hospital or healthcare system ownership.[23]

SUPPORTING URGENT CARE

To our knowledge, there are three national organizations dedicated to providing resources, education, and leadership for the urgent care practice of medicine. These include:

The Urgent Care Association of America (UCAOA) founded in 2004 (*www.ucaoa.org*)

The National Association for Ambulatory Care (NAFAC) founded in 1973 (*www.urgentcare.org*)

The Convenient Care Association (CCA) founded in 2006 (*www.ccaclinics.org*)

This list excludes professional practice associations with urgent care sections, including the American College of Emergency Physicians, American Academy of Family Physicians, American Association of Pediatrics, and the American College of Physicians.

During the past decade, retail urgent care clinics, also known as miniclinics or convenient care clinics, have also grown in popularity. These clinics are located in retail stores, such as Walgreens, CVS Caremark, and Walmart, and are focused on providing convenient access to care for minor medical conditions and immunizations. There are currently more than 1,000 retail medical clinics located in national pharmacy and grocery store chains.[24]

In addition, freestanding EDs—both hospital affiliated and private venture supported—are starting to appear in large urban areas. The American Hospital Association estimates that there are approximately 179 freestanding EDs, with the majority being hospital or healthcare system owned.[25]

WHAT PATIENTS WANT REGARDING NONEMERGENT CARE (BASED ON DEMOGRAPHICS)
1. **Young families** want care that is quick and available after hours.
2. **Young urban professionals (YUPPIE)** may be insured or uninsured but know that they have options in healthcare. They will discriminate based on price and convenience, and they have the resources to do so.
3. **Baby boomers** know what they want from healthcare providers. They are time and price conscious and will change providers for better, cheaper service.

Market competition plays a role in the development and expansion of both urgent care centers and freestanding EDs. Entrepreneur physicians and investors target markets capturing the insured population, similar to the boutique hospital competition for orthopedic, cardiovascular, and oncology services. Until now there have been limited choices for patients seeking access to immediate care, so by default hospitals have been receiving the revenue from paying patients for the treatment of minor ailments. Now, competition from urgent care centers can erode the patient population utilizing traditional hospitals for these services and result in financial struggles for these same hospitals. Healthcare executives should consider what the needs will be for the influx of newly insured Americans as a result of PPACA. Urgent care delivery models are one solution to providing cost-efficient medical care for those that are insured, on Medicaid, Medicare, or self-pay.

Defining Urgent Care Facilities

In general, an urgent care center is defined as:

The delivery of ambulatory care in a facility dedicated to the delivery of medical care outside of a hospital ED, usually on an unscheduled, walk-in basis. Urgent care centers are primarily used to treat patients who have an injury or illness that requires immediate care but is not serious enough to warrant a visit to an ED. Often urgent care centers are not open on a continuous basis, unlike a hospital ED, which would be open at all times.[26]

However, there is a mixed opinion among healthcare providers on what exactly constitutes an urgent care facility. For example, some healthcare professionals exclude retail medical and cash clinics from the definition of urgent care centers. We believe, however, that retail clinics are part of the entire spectrum of care and include these sites in our definition (see Figure 1.1 and Figure 1.2). We define urgent care facilities as follows.

Retail medical clinic: These sites are typically one or two rooms located in retail pharmacies, grocery stores, or chain stores. Staffing is a single provider, most often a nurse practitioner. These clinics are usually open during store hours, making visits convenient. They provide care for minor medical ailments, medical screening for cholesterol and diabetes, and provision of immunizations.

Cash clinic: These sites are commonly developed or sponsored by large healthcare organizations. They are most often cash only and provide a menu of options for care, including basic examinations, charge for additional lab work, and may perform minor procedures. They provide low-cost care for minor illnesses and

---

FIGURE 1.1

URGENT CARE SPECTRUM

Physician office	Routine care, chronic care, and health maintenance
Retail clinic/cash clinic	Minor illness care (sore throat, upper respiratory infection, urinary tract infections, and rashes), immunizations, and minor injuries (sprains, strains, and simple lacerations)
Moderate urgent care	Greater testing ability, waive testing, and care for the above illnesses, extends to more advanced injuries that require an x-ray
Advanced urgent care	Advanced injuries including fracture care, intravenous fluids therapy, repetitive dose aerosol breathing treatment, advanced diagnostics including computed tomography (CT) scans for evaluation of head injury, kidney stones and abdominal complaints
Freestanding ED	Care for all levels of injury—minor to advanced, typically exclude major trauma, may treat and stabilize all levels of medical care, typically include advanced imaging (CT, plain film radiography, ultrasound), full service lab
Acute care hospital	Care for all levels of illness and injury, including major trauma

---

injuries. Some have been developed as medical homes and are often staffed by nurse practitioners to maintain lower costs.

Urgent care center: These sites provide various levels of service, ranging from minor testing to complete labs and radiographic capability, approaching levels of an ED. Most centers are open extended hours, with some providing care 24 hours per day. They do not accept ambulance traffic and are most often staffed with

FIGURE 1.2

LEVELS OF URGENT CARE DEVELOPMENT

Basic level urgent care	Site with 1–3 beds: Limited waive testing, hours 8–12, with some weekend and afterhours component, (may be cash clinic or retail clinic)
Basic level urgent care	Site from 2–6 beds: Expanded waive testing, hours 8–12, with some weekend and afterhours component, no x-ray
Moderate level urgent care	Site from 6–10 beds: Expanded waive testing, hours 8–12, with some weekend and afterhours component, EKG, basic plain film x-ray
Moderate level urgent care	Site from 6–10 beds: Expanded waive testing, draw station with same day results, hours 12 or greater, with some weekend and afterhours component, basic plain film x-ray
Advanced level urgent care	Site from 6–10 beds: Waive testing with point of care blood tests, hours 12 or greater, with expanded weekend and afterhours component, EKG, basic plain film x-ray and CT scanning +/- ultrasound
Advanced level urgent care	Site from 6–10 beds: Expanded waive testing with point of care and on-site STAT lab (CBC, comprehensive metabolic, liver function tests), hours 16–24, open 7 days per week with afterhours component, EKG, radiology/Imaging center (plain films, ultrasound, CT scan)
	Freestanding emergency department

family practitioners, emergency physicians, nurse practitioners, physician assistants, or experienced internists.

Freestanding emergency departments: These sites provide all levels of care and stabilization, with the exception of those requiring major procedural interventions, such as a cardiac catheterization lab. Most freestanding EDs do not have the capability to admit patients but may provide extended observation for cases including gastroenteritis and asthma. They are usually hospital owned, but many recent centers have been private ventures supported by physicians.

The above definitions do not include free clinics or physician offices providing some urgent care services. In Chapter 2, we briefly discuss federally qualified healthcare clinics as a hybrid model under cash clinics. Our concept for this book was to avoid the medical home and focus on episodic care of illnesses and injuries.

ED and Urgent Care Interface

Urgent care centers are a potential source to decompress hospital EDs. ED visits continue to grow, with more than 123,000,000 patients in 2008, according to the Centers for Disease Control and Prevention (CDC). Many experts argue that up to one-third of these patients could be seen in other facilities; however, the American College of Emergency Physicians estimates that only 8% of these patients present for nonurgent medical care.[27] According to the CDC, only 12.1% of emergency visits are nonurgent and can be delayed or wait 2–24 hours for care. These statistics are significantly lower than the numbers espoused by the general media.

The majority of ED overcrowding is related to inpatients boarding in the ED.[28] The U.S. baby boomer population is aging, resulting in increased use of emergency services by geriatric patients with more complex medical histories that require longer and more detailed medical evaluation than younger patients. This patient group often requires hospitalization, further straining in patient hospital capacity. In the United States, there are approximately 5,800 registered acute care hospitals, with close to 950,000 hospital inpatient beds. Hospital inpatient capacity has also been significantly reduced as reimbursement changes occurred for inpatient care during the 1980s related to the Tax Equity and Fiscal Responsibility Act.[29]

Emergency departments are also affected by federal regulations for patient care unlike physician offices, private hospitals (not accepting Medicare or Medicaid), and clinics. Acute care hospitals that accept funding from Medicare and Medicaid programs are required by federal law through the Emergency Medical Treatment and Active Labor Act (EMTALA) to provide a medical screening exam and stabilizing treatment to any patient presenting to the facility with an emergency medical condition. If an emergency medical condition is not found, the patient may be referred to other facilities for care.

Given increased volumes of patients seeking treatment in EDs, strains on inpatient capacity, and the reduced number of hospital-based ED facilities, there is a vast opportunity for EDs and urgent care centers to work harmoniously to better deliver care to patients. The development of a strong relationship between the two types of facilities will be critical for smooth patient transitions. Depending on the level of care and staffing, most urgent care centers will need to transfer higher-level cases to the ED, for example patients with acute stroke symptoms. Likewise, to decrease utilization of the ED by nonemergent patient volume, many hospitals have developed screening programs that refer nonemergent cases out of the ED. In addition, urgent care centers can also serve as a temporary referral site for ED cases including wound checks, cellulitis rechecks, follow-up evaluation for musculoskeletal injuries, and follow-up evaluation from hospital discharge.

For example, Memorial Hermann Healthcare developed an ED screening program in 2003. The program uses nurse practitioners to screen patients with a set of clinical protocols and then refer patients without an emergency medical condition to a local cash clinic.[30] This clinic was supported and staffed by the healthcare system. In addition to these types of cash clinics, several hospitals are actively referring patients to local federally qualified healthcare centers after ED care has been provided. The desire is to reduce unnecessary ED visits for minor conditions.[31] These programs benefit the patient by providing a medical home, benefit the clinic with volume growth, benefit the hospital by alleviating overcrowding in the ED, and benefit the state by reducing healthcare costs.

By working more closely together, hospital EDs and urgent care centers can better provide the appropriate level of care to patients in the appropriate setting and potentially reduce healthcare costs. The goal should be for the right patient to be cared for at the right facility for the lowest cost.

REFERENCES

1. Censky, Annalyn. October jobs report: Unemployment rate dips. CNNMoney. Retrieved on 20 February 2012 from *http://money.cnn.com/2011/11/04/news/economy/jobs_report_unemployment/index.htm.*

2. Health United States. 2010. Retrieved 24 November 2011 from *www.cdc.gov/nchs/data/hus/hus10.pdf.*

3. The Kaiser Commission on Medicaid and the Uninsured. The Uninsured: A Primer. Retrieved on 20 June 2012 from *http://www.kff.org/uninsured/upload/7451-07.pdf.*

4. Jacobs, P., Rapoport, J. 2004. The Economics of Health and Medical Care. Jones and Burdett Publishers, Sadbury, MA.

5. American College of Emergency Physicians. 2011. Health Care Reform Fact Sheet. Retrieved 27 December 2011 from *www.acep.org/content.aspx?LinkIdentifier=id&id=45294&fid=3496&Mo=No&taxid=112443*.

6. Brophy, M. 2011. Study: Third of hospital ERs have closed over past 20 years. USA Today. Retrieved 20 December 2011 from *http://yourlife.usatoday.com*.

7. American College of Emergency Physicians. 2011. Health Care Reform Fact Sheet. Retrieved 27 December 2011 from *www.acep.org/content.aspx?LinkIdentifier=id&id=45294&fid=3496&Mo=No&taxid=112443*.

8. Williams, R.M. 1996. The Costs of Visits to Emergency Departments. N Engl J.Med. 334:642–646.

9. Ibid.

10. Krueger, Alan B., Kuziemko, Ilyana. The Demand for Health Insurance among Uninsured Americans: Results of a Survey Experiment and Implications for Policy. Princeton. Retrieved 19 June 2012 from *www.princeton.edu/~kuziemko/gallup_19june2011.pdf*.

11. Association of American Medical Colleges. The Impact of Health Care Reform on the Future Supply and Demand for Physicians Updated Projections Through 2025. Retrieved 19 June 2012 from *www.aamc.org/download/158076/data/updated_projections_through_2025.pdf*.

12. Health Reform Facts and Figures. Health Connector. Retrieved on 19 June 2012 from *www.mahealthconnector.org/portal/binary/com.epicentric.contentmanagement.servlet. ContentDeliveryServlet/Health%2520Care%2520Reform/Facts%2520and%2520Figures/ Facts%2520and%2520Figures.pdf*.

13. Smulowitz, P., Lipton, R., Wharman, F., et al. 2011. Emergency Department Utilization After Implementation of Massachusetts Health Reform. Ann Emerg Med. 58(3):225–233.

14. Long, S.K., Masi, P.B. 2009. Access and affordability: an update on health reform in Massachusetts, fall 2008. Health Aff. (Millwood). 28(4):w578–w587.

15. Massachusetts Medical Society Physician Workforce Study. September 2009.

16. ibid.

17. Zhu, J., Brwarsky, P., Lipsitz, S., Huskamp, Haas, J. 2010. Massachusetts Health Reform and Disparities in Coverage, Access, and Health Status. J Gen Intern Med. 25(12):1356–1362.

18. Kaiser.edu.org. Retrieved 20 May 2012 from w*ww.kaiseredu.org/Issue-Modules/Primary-Care-Shortage/Background-Brief.aspx.*

19. Weinick, R., Bristol, S., DesRoches, C. 2009. Urgent Care Centers in the U.S.: Findings from a National Survey. BMC Health Services Research. 9:79.

20. Kevinmd. 2011. Medicaid physician payment rates hurts primary care doctors. Retrieved 9 January 2012 from *www.kevinmd.com/blog/2010/04/medicaid-physician-payment-rates-hurts-primary-care-doctors.html.*

21. Center for Workforce Studies, Physician Shortages to Worsen without Increases in Residency Training. Association of American Medical Colleges. Retrieved 20 December 2011 from *www.aamc.org/download/150584/data/physician_shortages_factsheet.pdf.*

22. Ibid.

23. Urgent Care Association of America. 2011. Urgent Care Statistics and Benchmarking. Retrieved 20 December 2011 from *www.ucaoa.org/docs/UrgentCareMediaKit.pdf.*

24. Mehrotra, A., Hangsheng, L., et al. 2009. Comparing Costs and Quality of Care at Retail Clinics With That of Other Medical Settings for 3 Common Illnesses. Ann Intern Med 151(5):321-328.

25. Andrews, M. 2008. Need the emergency room? Skip the wait, hospital ERs have new competition: freestanding facilities that tout customer service. Retrieved December 2011 from *http://health.usnews.com/health-news/articles/2008/09/17/need-the-emergency-room-skip-the-wait.*

26. Wikipedia. Retrieved 20 May 2012 from *http://en.wikipedia.org/wiki/Urgent_care.*

27. American College of Emergency Physicians. 2011. Health Care Reform Fact Sheet. Retrieved 27 December 2011 from *www.acep.org/content.aspx?LinkIdentifier=id&id=45294&fid=3496&Mo=No& taxid=112443.*

28. Lucas, R., Parley, H., Twanmoh, J., et al. Measuring the Opportunity Loss of Time Spent Boarding Admitted Patients in the Emergency Department: A Multihospital Analysis. Journal of Healthcare Management. 54(2):117-125.

29. Smith, D., Pickard, R. 1986 Evaluation of the Impact of Medicare and Medicaid prospective payment on Utilization of Philadephia Area Hospitals. Health Serv Res. 21(4):529–546.

30. Jaklevic, M. 2003. All Cash. All the Time. Modern Healthcare. 33(25):40.

31. Tull, K. 2010. Grant helps ED refer patients to health center. ED Management: The Monthly Update on Emergency Department Management. 22(3):29–31.

Affiliation and Ownership

Hospital and healthcare systems compete daily for patient volumes from boutique hospitals, such as heart hospitals, and independently owned clinics. Several states may require a certificate of need for additional acute care beds, including those in hospital-owned urgent care centers. Still, there are many reasons that hospitals or health systems may want to develop freestanding urgent care centers, including decompression of a currently stressed emergency department (ED), protecting current business and location from competition, developing a new geographic territory, and improving current financial demographics by targeting specific communities.[1]

Business Case

As inpatient revenue continues to decrease, it is critical to expand outpatient services for the viability of the healthcare system. Having a robust outpatient growth strategy can help preserve market share. Hospital administrators should be aware of these types of opportunities. For example, many patients will seek the most cost-effective alternative when he or she is responsible for the majority of the out-of-pocket costs. In addition to costs, young professionals also consider time as potential capital and will gravitate to the fastest modality that provides services for the healthcare need—and that may not be your hospital.

Loss of revenue

Although healthcare executives may complain that urgent care centers receive lower levels of reimbursement, these facilities do provide substantial revenue when added together. Consider an ED that isn't treating sore throats, minor lacerations, and ankle sprains, among other nonemergent conditions. There would be a great deal more idle time. Three minor ankle sprains often generate more revenue than one critical care patient. Loss of this revenue may be a major issue for hospitals.

Even low-acuity patients are sources of revenue. Hospitals and other entities should take notice of their retail clinic competition and the reduced costs of care for minor medical complaints. These sites are becoming much more competitive for minor complaints and often provide care for costs lower than the local physician office, urgent care facility, and ED on a per-visit basis.[2,3]

In addition, insurance carriers are actively pursuing strategies to educate consumers regarding where to seek treatment to reduce ED visits for low-acuity complaints. Anthem Blue Cross and Blue Shield of Virginia, for example, reduced ED visits by 14% through an educational campaign. Its program combined online e-mail education, financial incentives by reducing copays from $10–$40 dollars for urgent care clinic use compared to copays of $100–$200 for ED visits, and providing information on local clinics via websites that incorporated the Google Maps program to provide locations of available clinics.[4] Administrators should be aware of these types of initiatives in their community that may result in significant loss of revenue, and health systems can prevent this market share erosion by constructing or developing a facility-owned urgent care center.

FIVE REASONS FOR A CEO TO OPEN A FREESTANDING URGENT CARE CENTER

1. **Securing the borders.** Developing an urgent care center before the competition does.

2. **Planting the flag.** Venturing into new territory of a competitor or growing area in need of healthcare services. It could also be the first step for a new hospital site.

3. **Helping the ED.** Helping to off-load some of the lower-acuity patients from the ED.

4. **Improving the ED payer mix.** Developing a cash clinic to refer ED patients to.

5. **Appealing to another patient population.** Offering faster services and lower costs.

Urgent Care Models

Rather than constructing a new ED, the hospital or health system CEO may consider adding inpatient beds and building an off-site urgent care center. This not only helps decongest the ED but also prevents loss of market share. If the new urgent care site is strategically located, it may bring in more referral business from an untapped competitor's market. Construction costs may also be lower for an off site urgent care center than a new ED—especially if any current demolition on the hospital site would be required.

Hospital affiliated

Hospital-affiliated clinics often have greater access to capital and the ability to combine other services, including a complete imaging center (discussed in Chapter 7). The imaging center and urgent care center tend to comarket each other and increase volume. For example, patients coming for an outpatient radiology test may realize the site also offers afterhours medical care. Similarly, the urgent care center becomes the major customer of the imaging center.

The ideal size for these sites ranges from 3,000–3,500 square feet or larger, with 6–10 beds that can easily provide care for 60–80 patients in a 12-hour period. Urgent care center staffing would require a minimum of one registration person, two or three registered nurses (if budgetary issues are present, this could be substituted with a licensed two-year degree program nurse), one medical technician, a nurse practitioner or physician assistant, and a physician. The professional component covering the nurse practitioner, physician assistant, and physician may be employed by the hospital, included in a joint venture, or contracted.

Our experience is most extensive with the last model. In the contracted model, the provider may be paid a set fee for services by the facility or bill patients directly for services. Depending on the level of staffing, additional stipends may be required to be paid by the hospital to the contractor when direct patient billing does not cover the costs of the requested staffing.

Income is directly related to volume and flow. We believe that each bed should turn over three to four times per hour at maximum flow, depending on the acuity of the patient and staffing of the site. Service capabilities vary by site but often include a minimum of Clinical Laboratory Improvement Amendment–waived testing and plain film x-ray capability. More comprehensive sites include a full-service lab and imaging center. Depending on where your facility is located, the hospital-affiliated clinic may require a certificate of need from the state before even considering development of an urgent care center.

CERTIFICATE-OF-NEED STATES	
Alabama	New Jersey
Alaska	New York
Arkansas	North Carolina
Georgia	South Carolina
Hawaii	Tennessee
Kentucky	Vermont
Maryland	Washington
Mississippi	West Virginia
Montana	District of Columbia

Retail clinic

Examples of commercially owned urgent care centers are MinuteClinic and RediClinic. The space requirements for these clinics range from 200–400 square feet, with one or two exam rooms located in a local pharmacy or grocery store chain. Staffing is a single provider—usually a nurse practitioner due to the ability for independent practice. These sites often have kiosk registration portals. Insurance cards and licenses are scanned into an automated system by the provider. There are a limited number of services at these sites including treatment for minor illnesses and injuries, as well as receiving physical examinations and immunizations. These sites often have an electronic medical record (EMR) with templates for all the minor care ailments it treats (e.g., sore throat, rash, upper respiratory infection, etc.), making data entry simple. Portions of the EMR may be electronically forwarded to the patient's primary care provider in a Healthcare Insurance Portability and Accountability Act of 1996–compliant fashion. The provider works under a well-defined protocol with telephone oversight available, in addition to immediate referral to other facilities for more advanced care. Although most of these clinics are commercially owned by each specific retailer, the business model is solid and could be accomplished by a healthcare system or individual entrepreneur working with a retailer in a joint venture or through lease space.

Cash clinics

These sites are typically owned or sponsored by large healthcare systems or communities. Most often they are small with only four to six beds. Staffing includes a receptionist, medical technician, nurse, and midlevel provider. Visits are charged on a sliding scale based on acuity, level of care provided, procedures, and ancillary tests. Many of these sites are set up to become medical homes for patients with chronic diseases, including diabetes, hypertension, and asthma/chronic obstructive pulmonary disease. In addition, they provide episodic care for minor injuries, such as simple laceration repair, incision and drainage of abscess, and minor illness, such as upper respiratory infections, sore throat, and urinary tract infections.

Location is critical for these sites. They should be in close proximity to the clienteles' neighborhood. Costs can be lower by leasing space in a local strip mall rather than building a stand-alone center. In addition, close proximity to a major medical center provides an instant referral base both from the local ED and, in more acute cases, to the ED.

Federally qualified community health centers

As referred to in the previous section, federally qualified community health centers are focused on providing care for the indigent and Medicaid populations. They accept Medicaid and those with insufficient resources for healthcare. Services are often billed on a sliding scale based on the patient's ability to pay. These centers do provide urgent care services but are usually more oriented toward a medical home model, focused on managing chronic conditions. Support for these centers is through a combination of federal and community funds with various levels of staffing and capability. Many sites include dental care, mental health counseling, and medical care. Some have medication on site that they can dispense at lower prices, as well. These centers can be an alternative to a hospital developing a cash clinic. Hospitals should ideally partner with these sites to increase volume for the clinic and decrease unnecessary visits to the ED, so the partnership or affiliation benefits both parties.[5]

Independent Urgent Care Models

As discussed in Chapter 1, the majority of urgent care centers are independently owned by physicians or physician groups. The first step to establish a clinic under this model is to understand the state's laws and potential licensing requirements for urgent care centers. As of January 2012, Arizona is the only state that requires licensing for urgent care centers. Several states, including Texas, California, Ohio,

Colorado, Iowa, Illinois, New York, and New Jersey, maintain laws regarding corporate practice of medicine. Simply stated, you must be a physician and have a physician license to operate a center where this law is in place. You should investigate your state and local requirements before opening any business. Obviously, most municipalities require some type of local business license.

The second step in the process is determining funding for the business venture. Obviously, space, staff, equipment, and supplies are required unless the plan involves investing in a franchise package or existing office space. Details for all these aspects are discussed at length in later chapters. Salaries for the first three to six months may need to be funded. There are significant delays in private insurance, Medicaid, Medicare participation agreements, and obtaining specific provider numbers for billing purposes. In addition, the nature of insurance is often to have payment delays exceeding 60–90 days. One consideration is to initially start with a "cash-only" policy and work toward accepting insurance plans. This may reduce startup costs; however, it may also reduce patient traffic due to out-of-pocket expense and the need for individuals to file insurance claims themselves. Medicare participation and provider numbers can take more than 90 days, and retroactive reimbursement is limited. You may consider delaying acceptance of Medicare billing until after provider numbers have been received and opt for cash payment.

Location is key to success. If this is a for-profit venture, the location should be in a high-traffic area near malls to improve volume. In addition, the review of local demographic data, including average housing prices, employment, and average family income levels, can help augment your ability to locate the facility in areas with a better payer mix. Locating your site near large medical facilities provides "spill-over" business that benefits your service by marketing turnaround better than that of the local ED. Medical office condos are an option but are likely higher priced, and you may have significant competition from other providers.

Finally, the size of the facility will depend on projected volume and the desire for growth. Most urgent care centers evaluate 30–60 patients per day, which can be handled with as few as six beds depending on flow. Determining which ancillary services to include, such as lab and radiology testing, are discussed in Chapter 7.

There has been a significant increase in the number of combined urgent care clinics and imaging centers. These are high-dollar operations and typically require hospital system backing or a joint venture with a large radiology group. Urgent care centers benefit greatly from plain film radiography and CT scanning that can expand the acuity level and type of medical condition treated. In addition, the imaging center benefits from the urgent care center's patient traffic with return visits occurring from previous urgent care patients for services, including mammograms and bone density testing at the imaging center.

There are many different models for urgent care center ownership and affiliation. The initial goal for the center will lead planners to the appropriate size, location, financing, marketing, facility, and equipment. Determining which model to choose ties back to the original intent of the urgent care center's mission to treat indigent patients versus insured and very-low-acuity versus more complex patients.

Chapter 2

REFERENCES

1. Craig, T. 1986. An Initial Marketing/Financial Screen Multiprogram Urgent Care Center. J Health Care Market. 6(4):61–73.

2. Mehrotra, A., Hangsheng, L., et al. 2009. Comparing Costs and Quality of Care at Retail Clinics with That of Other Medical Settings for 3 Common Illnesses. Ann Intern Med 151(5):321-329.

3. Bowling, K. 2011. Health Care Goes Retail, Solantic Looks to Retail Marketing Models to Strengthen Its Brand. Market Health Serv. 3(2):20.

4. Wellpoint. 23 June 2011. Emergency Room Interventions Using Google Maps and Education Empower Consumers to Choose ER Alternatives for Nonemergency Conditions. Retrieved 17 December 2011 from *http://ir.wellpoint.com/phoenix.zhtml?c=130104&p=irol-newsArticle& ID=1579424&highlight.*

5. Sorelle, R. August 2011. Community Health Centers Ease ED's Burden. Emergency Medicine News P6.

Creating a Financial Plan

Planning an urgent care center should be done with careful consideration of the clientele who will be served, anticipated patient volume, and any special needs the patients and families may have. Financing for urgent care centers may come from a hospital or healthcare system, joint venture, physician group or partnership, or a single physician. Although hospitals can finance urgent care sites with existing capital, physicians often must find startup capital from their own personal finances (e.g., home equity, cash on hand, or investments) or borrow the funds from banks or other lenders.

Market Considerations

Once the decision has been made to pursue development of an urgent care center, the following questions will help guide the planning process and help define the best fit from a facility and financing prospective.

1. What market share will be served?

    •   Age of patients (consider breaking this into the following three groups: under 18 years of age, 18–55 years of age, and over the age of 55)

- What are the projected payers for these patient groups?

- What are the injury and illness profiles that will drive services for each one of these patient populations?

2. Who are the competitors currently providing services to this market?

  - Which emergency departments?

  - Which competing urgent care centers?

  - Which primary care practices?

3. Which of these competitors can support or collaborate with the urgent care center being developed? For example, the urgent care center agrees to provide after hours backup for local pediatricians.

Financing 101

Whether the site is to be hospital affiliated, owned, a joint venture, or developed by a physicians or a physician group, you will need to construct a basic financial plan and proforma. In general, an urgent care center that will see between 12,000 to 16,000 visits annually can operate efficiently in 2,500–4,000 square feet. Once volume figures are ascertained, staffing can be projected based on the average number of arrivals and appropriate benchmarks (see Chapter 6). These figures enable you to plan for the number of exam rooms, types of testing, and size of waiting areas that will be needed. All these costs need to be determined to develop a financial plan and proforma.

The wise clinic owner will do his or her homework and answer these questions before any leases are signed or buildings are purchased. The proforma is then presented to hospital executives in the case of hospital ownership or joint venture for approval of financing or to the bank or other lending institutions if funded by a physician or physician groups.

Capital required

We project that the capital required for starting an urgent care clinic ranges from $500,000–$800,000. In addition, you will likely need a credit line for the first year to fund payroll, as "break even" financial performance requires several months to a year to establish. This is due to the time required for volume to grow, delays in attaining credentialing through various managed care organization carriers and Medicare, and the typical delays in accounts receivable for patient billing payments from various insurance products. A poorly planned clinic often runs short on capital in the first year, resulting in closure and potential bankruptcy.

Due to the current interest rate climate, funding in 2012 is relatively lower cost than in years past. Securing funding of $1 million or less can often be accomplished through a local bank. If you are expanding and seek capital of $5 million or greater to fund multiple clinics, you may consider a partnership with another corporation with greater capital assets, subordinated debt, or approach equity investors. The latter can be arranged privately or through your local investment banker.

Funding sources

As we have discussed regarding recent healthcare reform regulations, private equity firms have began investing heavily in urgent care sites in the belief that significant volume and financial opportunity exist. The point is that the market has recently shifted due to this new influx of funding. Both physicians and hospitals need to understand that in specific geographic markets, multiple urgent care sites will be coming in the near future. Whether these new urgent care sites are funded and controlled by a private physician or hospital competition, they will be coming from other private sources.

Financial sources for independent providers may be from personal assets, bank loans, subordinated debt, equity investors, or hospital joint ventures. The cost of capital is tied to the amount required, collateral available, and potential profit of the site. One of the most important planning components is the retention and use of legal counsel with healthcare experience and ensuring that you have your own accountant as part of the team that is assessing all of the financing options available.

Investment bankers can introduce you to private equity investors who will perform significant due diligence and require documentation of clinic performance, proforma/EBITA detail, corporate structure and governance, current and past malpractice history, and even personal financial data. Obviously, most investors will want to be involved in the financial management of the clinic and be involved in any purchase of additional sites or sale of existing sites.

Franchise opportunities are also available to physicians and provide turn-key operations with assistance determining the location, staffing, supply and equipment purchase, and other consulting advice. Franchise programs should be

---

FIGURE 3.1

HEALTHCARE FRANCHISE RESOURCES

Legal considerations:[1]
- Corporate practice of medicine and anti-fee splitting statute
- Joint ventures, management arrangements, and service agreements
- Implication of anti-kickback statutes

Franchise opportunities:
- HealthcareFranchises.net *(www.HealthcareFranchises.net)*
- MedHelp Urgent Care *(www.urgentcareatlanta.com/franchise.html)*

---

aware of the state laws regarding corporate practice of medicine that require only licensed healthcare professionals or professional healthcare organizations to provide healthcare services (see Figure 3.1). In addition, laws pertaining to billing and fee splitting make it illegal for income from patient care to be shared with anyone (including a corporation) other than the entity or organization providing the care.

Key Takeaway

Financial analysis and proforma development are required to ensure that the urgent care clinic is worth consideration as a viable opportunity. Funding may come from hospital capital, banking, other debt, or private equity. Private equity funding has dramatically increased recently, backing many of the larger urgent care vendors, which has resulted in a significant increase of competition in certain geographic markets.

Chapter 3

REFERENCE

1. Can You Franchise an Urgent Care Concept? Retrieved 27 December 2011 from *www.franchise lawsolutions.com/library/health-law-attorney-new-york-franchising-and-urgent-care-center.cfm.*

Facility Considerations

The largest initial expense for an urgent care center is typically the building. Several aspects are important to the selection of the site, including location, size, and internal construction costs. Once the location is decided, the decision regarding lease versus purchase is required. Finally, the internal components of the facility, including space allocation and equipment, need to be determined. In short, there are five basic facility questions that need to be asked.

- What is the best location for an urgent care center?

- Should the property be purchased or leased?

- What are the positives and negatives of leasing versus buying?

- How much space will the clinic need?

- What basic equipment will be needed for the urgent care center?

Location Is Crucial

The real estate mantra "location, location, location" is right on target when it comes to urgent care centers. The location of your urgent care site will often mean the difference between success and failure. It is imperative to do your due diligence and complete your homework on location results.

The premarketing plan should determine a location that is highly traveled, visible from the street, and has ample parking. Depending on the intent of the facility—an indigent care clinic versus a for-profit site—local employment information, housing costs, and foreclosure data can assist you in identifying the best site. You also should perform a detailed evaluation of local competitors, including other urgent care centers, primary care physician practices, and hospital emergency departments (ED).

The catchment area should have a service population of greater than 25,000 within five square miles, with an ideal population being around 50,000. Road traffic volume should exceed 25,000 vehicles along the facing street of the facility, similar to data suggested by National UC Realty *(www.nationalucr.com)*. Commuters should be able to see your large "Urgent Care" signage during the day and night (make sure it is well lit in the evening). One note of caution: You need to know what each state's laws are for signage and the description of your center, because some states do not allow the title of "Urgent Care" to be used. In addition, you should have your corporate attorney (a required person that owners and organizations need) ensure that your urgent care center name is not already trademarked. This will prevent later disasters requiring name changes and renegotiation of all contracts, including managed care under the new name if the managed care contract is listed under the facility rather than the provider.

Target demographic

Local population demographics, including household size, average age, and per-capita income, can be obtained from your municipality or United States census data. Information may also be available from local healthcare facilities regarding payer mix in the region that will assist you in identifying the correct target population. Patient volume can be approximated by estimating visits based on the demographic group obtained from the Centers for Disease Control and Prevention (CDC). The CDC provides information on utilization by age and payer class. Local realtors can provide a wealth of information regarding home sales, foreclosures, and average home costs. These estimates are general in nature, and accuracy can be very challenging when other healthcare providers are located in the same area. Higher volume and market development can be accomplished in areas with limited healthcare penetration, located near major retail shopping, and in close proximity to neighborhoods with younger families. Young families also provide for long-term growth opportunities. Further information and assistance can be obtained through commercial firms including National UC Realty (*http://nationalucr.com/*). Its research is the basis for some of the information listed under the sidebar "Demographics for Success."

DEMOGRAPHICS FOR SUCCESS

5 mile radius: 25,000–50,000 population

Median income: >50,000

Close to retail stores: Restaurant chains, grocery stores, and pharmacies

---

If the site is going to be hospital owned or affiliated with a healthcare organization, preplanning should identify areas where current staff physicians have offices to reduce perceptions of competition with hospital-affiliated medical staff. Many physicians consider medical office condos as an ideal location for urgent care centers. But in our opinion, this choice often does not provide the patient volume required for success, unless the site is specifically designated as the urgent care center for a large multispecialty practice. Once an office is established, maintaining the same location will help build an established clientele.

Location and size

The purpose of the urgent care clinic determines the size needed and the ideal location required. See Figure 4.1 for a description of the types of urgent care centers and their location and size requirements. The space requirement depends on the intent of the site and complexity of its care. It can range from a single treatment room with an examining bed at a retail clinic to a complete freestanding ED. Larger space results in greater fixed costs, requiring increased revenue and patient volume to cover these costs.

FIGURE 4.1

URGENT CARE CLINIC SIZE ESTIMATES

TYPE	BEDS	ESTIMATED SQUARE FOOTAGE
Retail clinic	1–2	< 400
Cash clinic	4–5	< 3,000
Urgent care	5–10	3,500–10,000
Freestanding ED	10–14	> 10,000

Convenient parking is essential, and it should be easily accessible from the roadway. Suggested parking requirements are five or more spaces per 1,000 square feet of medical office space. Dedicated parking for the site enables easier access to the clinic, especially for those patients who have difficulty walking due to illness, age, or injury. The front office staff should be keenly aware of arriving patients in order to provide wheelchair assistance when needed.

Retail clinics require minimal square footage and are usually located in retail pharmacies or grocery stores or other retail complexes.

Cash clinic developers should consider locations on major metro bus or subway lines to make access easier for patients without private modes of transportation. In addition, locating the site near a large healthcare facility will provide for an automatic referral base from that facility's ED. Selecting sites in a local strip mall close to the targeted population or neighborhood can also help increase traffic and utilization. Cash clinics require moderate square footage of less than 3,000 square feet.

Commercial or hospital-based urgent care centers are larger and often located in high-traffic areas close to local shopping with ample parking and ease of access. Access and signage are critical for these sites to be successful. The clinic signage should be easily visible from the entrance roadway as well as highways that are in close proximity. The "open" sign should be well lit, providing easy visibility during evening hours. In addition, digital signage (e.g., light-emitting diode or liquid crystal display) should be considered, because it captures the eye of local vehicle and pedestrian traffic. Digital messages can be easily varied to promote products, services, and healthcare information.

In general, urgent care clinics treat 12,000–16,000 patients annually and operate efficiently in about 2,500–3,000 square feet.

Lease vs. Ownership

Given the depressed real estate economy the United States is currently experiencing in most urban and rural areas, it is recommended that leasing space be considered at least during the startup and practice development period of the urgent care center life cycle. This is a cost-effective solution for getting the business up and running as well as allowing the business accounts receivable to grow. This strategy helps the business substantiate revenue growth and improve borrowing power.

The decision to lease versus purchase the space is based on current cash available, market conditions, and suitable locations available. If credit is an issue or if there is limited capital available for the startup, leasing requires less qualification. Hospitals and healthcare systems usually have fewer issues in obtaining capital than independent physician practices. Leasing provides the tax benefit of being 100% deductible but includes no ownership or site appreciation benefit. Lease costs are variable, averaging about $20 per square foot, with additional charges for common area management that can add $3–$6 per square foot. It may be wise to start with a smaller space with room to grow as volumes increase. Leasing may also allow expansion into adjacent space as the site grows or relocation to a better area once the lease has ended.

Structural changes are often at the cost of the leaser, with room construction and internal modifications starting at $75 per square foot. Negotiation with the owner may yield positive results with shared construction costs under a tenant improvement allowance. Build-out and modification of lease space often requires 90 days or more to complete unless the space was a previous medical office.

Risks of leasing include potential problems with adjacent tenants and foreclosure of the owner, especially with many partially occupied strip malls. You should consider clauses including "subordination and non disturbance" requiring the new owner to continue leasing without business disturbance of the urgent care site. Parking may also be an issue if other tenants monopolize the space. In addition, lease agreements should have an option for renewal to avoid business interruption and prevent the need for relocation. Having the first right refusal to purchase allows you to be the first person in line to purchase the property if it goes on the market. You need to have a qualified attorney review the lease agreement to avoid later problems.

There are many vacant video store sites available for lease or purchase. These sites average between 6,000–10,000 square feet and are ideal for a 10-bed urgent care site with a plain film room and waive testing lab. Larger sites could accommodate CT scanning facilities, as well. Our review revealed that these properties were available for purchase ranging from $130–$350 per square foot. The costs for an adequate location likely starts at $1.5 million, if purchased, resulting in a monthly mortgage close to $10,000 depending on money down and the loan interest rate. The most critical aspect for your site is that you do not overbuild or pick a site that is too large. Most urgent care clinics average around 3,000 square feet.

REASONS TO PURCHASE VS. LEASE
• Historically low interest rates
• Vacant strip mall space/video stores
• Small Business Administration backing with as little as 10% down
• Real estate appreciation
• Tax-advantaged depreciation
• If leasing a multiunit facility, you cannot control the behavior of others

Defining Internal Spaces

Whether the site is purchased or leased, internal design is often required unless it was previously a medical office clinic. Many aspects of healthcare design are regulated by local, state, and federal codes. It is important to consult with a medical architect who can assist you and ensure that these code requirements are met. In addition the architect can be of significant value in designing improved work flow for staff.

The American College of Emergency Physicians produced a guide, *Emergency Department Design: A Practical Guide for the Future,* that is a great source regarding space requirements and design basics; however, some modification is required for urgent care centers.[1] Many of our suggested specifications are based on this publication. In addition, the American Institute of Architects publishes *Guidelines for Design and Construction of Hospital and Health Care Facilities,* which can also be an excellent reference tool. The most critical aspect is the use of a qualified architect to assist in the site design so that your site is functional, compliant, and welcoming.

Volume figures can be used to determine the number of exam rooms and the sizes of testing/storage spaces and waiting areas. It is crucial that the urgent care center functions in an efficient and highly regimented fashion, characterized only by forward progress after registration and insurance verification and copayment processes are completed.

Important aspects to remember, whether it's a new construction or an internal retrofit, include installing an appropriate power supply and structural support for procedure lights and radiology equipment and adequate electrical outlets and cabinet and counter space in exam rooms and nurse/provider stations. Also consider installing sinks in each treatment room, even though plumbing can be very expensive.

The following breaks down design principles for the required areas in your urgent care center.

Waiting area

Your waiting room (approximately 400 square feet) should be clean, spacious, and welcoming. The front entrance should have an automatic double door or a large single door that can easily provide access for a large wheelchair and an ambulance stretcher. The waiting room should have at least two to three chairs per examination room with 12–15 square feet per chair. In addition, you will require at least one unisex restroom that is disability accessible; the size is often specified by local code. The waiting area likely will require a minimum of 400–500 square feet for an 8–10-room urgent care center. You should also consider installing free WiFi and a large plasma screen television to improve patient experience.

Registration area

The registration area (approximately 200 square feet) should have ample space for a computer/printer, credit card acceptance device, scanner for license and insurance submission, compliant paper shredder (or shred bin), and a safe for cash collections. The site should have an advanced phone system that can handle multiple calls with prerecorded menu options. Although many people dislike these prerecorded programs, the site should use the service for providing detailed directions to its location(s), office hours, and types of service provided (e.g., injury, illness, occupational medicine, immunizations, travel services, etc.). The phone system with prerecorded messages can free up your registration personnel from prolonged conversations on directions and office hours, allowing them to focus on incoming patients and obtaining accurate registration information. At least one registration booth is required, but space for two is suggested to allow for peak-volume registration and future growth.

Triage

Some smaller facilities may not need triage. A triage area (100 square feet) is designated for rapid evaluation and sorting of higher- versus lower-acuity patients and should be used only when treatment rooms are full. The goal should be immediate bedding, placing the patient directly in a treatment room upon arrival; this practice helps improve patient satisfaction with the visit. The standard triage room includes a small desk and chair for nursing staff to document information and should include a computer for sites with electronic health records. The patient also requires a chair. Equipment placed in the room includes a vital-sign device (preferably automated), infant scale, adult scale, thermometer, and minor wound care supplies.

Treatment rooms

Patient preference strongly suggests the use of all private rooms (approximately 100–120 square feet per room). Many doctor's offices have exam rooms averaging 100 square feet (10 ft by 10 ft). This space provides for a single visitor's chair, physician or provider stool, small desk with sink and upper cabinetry, and a short examination table. The short examination table allows for an adequate exam and has storage space below the table, and paper coverings can be used instead of sheets, which can reduce the cost of laundry and speed up the bed turnover process. These beds are often $1,000 each, compared to the traditional ED stretcher, costing upward of $5,000. Obviously, the room size may be expanded based on desire, but most minor complaints can be cared for in a room of this size.

Procedure rooms

Most urgent care centers perform multiple procedures, including laceration repairs, incision and drainage, and casting and splinting, among others. These procedures require more space and a comfortable, recumbent patient. We recommend at least one procedure room (approximately 144 square feet). With a volume of more than 40 patients per day, you could easily justify a second procedure room. The rooms are often 144 square feet (12 ft by 12 ft) or larger to allow for a full-size stretcher. Obviously, the stretcher needs to easily transit the door space when you need to take the patient for x-rays or additional diagnostic tests. The room should contain all necessary equipment (secured access to prevent theft), including suture sets, incision and drainage trays, splinting equipment, etc. Lighting is also important, and either a portable spotlight for procedures or an overhead surgical light is required. The portable spotlight is mobile, less expensive, and could be utilized in other rooms.

Restroom

The number of restrooms and square footage requirements (accessible, approximately 100 square feet per room) are likely spelled out in local code. For most urgent care clinics, we suggest at least three restrooms, with one in the waiting area, one in the treatment area, and one for staff (that could be shared). The restroom design is critical if drug screenings are to be done, which require the toilet area to be isolated away from running water and the ability to externally adjust the flushing mechanism (turn off).[2] These items are necessary to prevent adulteration of specimens and require a door between the toilet and the sink.

Nurse/provider area

The nurse's station and provider area (approximately 300–400 square feet) allocates space for documentation, communication, and management of the clinic. It is crucial that most of the treatment area is visible from this central station. Depending on your site, this area may need space for a waive testing lab, picture archiving and communication system (PACS), or radiology review area, as well as a medication preparation and dispensing area that is free from interruption to avoid medication errors. Patient care documentation occurs either at the bedside or in this central area, requiring at least space for three computer workstations (one for the physician, one for the nurse, and one for the unit secretary/technician/additional provider). We would hope that each site has a computer-based medical record and tracking system, especially for larger sites. In addition, the station should have multiple phone lines along with at least two or three phones to assist in communication.

Breakroom

The staff requires an "off stage" area to take breaks (approximately 150–200 square feet). The Occupational Safety and Health Administration (OSHA) also requires that any food consumption be completely separate from treatment areas. The room must be enclosed, i.e., have a door, to prevent blood exposure or other contamination. Adequate space would include room for a table with chairs, microwave, refrigerator (for staff food only), and a flat-screen television. This is an ideal area to post information for staff, required employment/OSHA information, etc.

Storage/utility rooms

Urgent care sites require adequate space (approximately 100–300 square feet) for supplies such as crutches, suture sets, and splints. In addition, codes may require both clean and soiled utility areas. One critical concept is that medical waste needs to be disposed of safely and following regulations to prevent injury of staff, patients, and anyone handling the material, especially sharps, including needles and scalpels.

Equipment and Supply Needs

The second significant startup cost for urgent care centers is the equipment costs. Capital expenditures will include computers and necessary telecommunication devices both for the office practice and for the electronic registration, coding, and billing submission. In addition, capital items include the exam room equipment and necessary point-of-care laboratory testing equipment (most of which is actually supplied by the laboratory vendors), and, if the center will do radiographic testing, the x-ray equipment. Please refer to Appendix A for more specifics on required facility equipment.

Urgent care clinics also require a wide variety of replaceable supplies, from Band-Aids to knee immobilizers, as well as standard equipment. Most equipment and supplies are available through major medical supply companies. These companies provide one-stop shopping in an effort to provide competitive prices and bulk purchasing. Common questions administrators have regarding supplies include the following:

- Where do I get clinic equipment and supplies?

- How should I track patient use or supplies and charges?

- What drugs should I keep in stock?

- Should we dispense complete prescriptions or only a single dose of medication along with a written prescription?

Purchasing supplies and equipment

Urgent care equipment and supplies can be purchased new or refurbished, and there are brand-name and generic options. Brand loyalty for specific pieces of equipment may be surprisingly more expensive than buying the generic version. You do not need to be brand loyal when you are purchasing supplies and equipment. In fact, many higher-cost items can be purchased either refurbished or with minor cosmetic defects that still function without problems. Likewise, generic options may work just as well as the higher-cost brand-name version.

These supplies need to be readily available, and all inventory needs to be maintained to run a successful urgent care clinic. Close tracking of patient use helps prevent lost charges, as well (see Example Patient Charge Master in Appendix D).

Basic equipment needs can be obtained from medical suppliers and include stretchers, exam tables, lighting, ophthalmoscopes, etc. These equipment needs are described in the following text. Being prepared for emergencies is critical, and urgent care sites should have a fully stocked "code" or resuscitation cart. In addition, we suggest that at minimum sites include adult and pediatric bag/mask setups, basic airway equipment (oral airways), and an automated external defibrillator. There are newer devices that can provide defibrillation, 12-lead capability, and cardiac/pulse oximetry monitoring, but keep in mind that these devices may require higher levels of training.

Patient supplies can be bought in bulk at lower prices, but make sure items that expire are closely monitored to avoid waste. Bandages, ace wraps, and splints obviously do not expire, but you should make sure that charges are not missed, resulting in financial loss for the facility. In our opinion, medication and supply management devices provide automatic patient charges, improve patient safety, and assist with inventory control by improving clinic revenue and reducing costs.

Disposable versus reusable equipment pits convenience against cost savings. The two most common procedures in our clinics are suturing of wounds and drainage of abscesses. With a volume of about 1,800–2,000 patients per month, we average approximately 100 laceration repairs and 30–40 abscess drainage procedures.

The required equipment for laceration repair includes a needle driver, forceps/tweezers, various clamps, skin hooks, and scissors (or scalpel). These can be purchased as reusable components for approximately $150 per set (we suggest you would need at least three sets) along with an autoclave for sterilization at a cost of less than $1,000. The supplies needed for incision and drainage include a scalpel, forceps, and clamps. Drapes and packing are best purchased as single-use items.

Many urgent care sites have shifted to disposable suture sets and incision/drainage packs due to ease and speed of preparation. But we have found that some of the instruments in these disposal sets are poor quality, especially needle holders.

We advise that you perform your own cost analysis to evaluate whether disposable or reusable supplies are the most appropriate for your site.

A medical supply vendor can provide recommendations and help explain the differences between various products to help you determine which supplies are the most cost-effective choices for your practice. (Please see Appendix B: Example Supply Inventory List).

Pharmaceutical needs

Urgent care clinics require a basic set of medications for patient use while patients are undergoing care on-site. Many patients will require immunizations, as well as prescriptions to treat infections, pain, and other conditions. Each site will need to determine whether advanced treatment, including intravenous (IV) fluids, nebulizer treatments, and IV antibiotics will be done by the clinic. As with supplies, it is vital that pharmaceuticals are closely managed to ensure patient safety, avoid issues with patient allergies and medication interactions, and minimize losses from medication expiration and lost income from poor control of inventory (lost patient charges). Medication management systems can help centers monitor pharmaceuticals.

The basic medications provided by most urgent care clinics include acetamino-phen, salycilates, and antinausea medication. (A suggested minimum medication list is included in Appendix C.)

Tetanus immunizations are frequently required after injuries, as well. In addition, immunization programs may be profitable by expanding the types of immuniza-tions offered to include hepatitis A, hepatitis B, influenza, and other immunizations.

More than half of clinic patient visits receive prescription medications. But it can be challenging for patients to fill prescriptions afterhours, so many patients will wait until the next day to get their prescription filled and start their medication. One option to address this challenge is that urgent care clinics may provide the first dose and expect that the patient fills the prescription the next day. Providing the entire prescription to the patient could also be an option, but pharmaceuticals are often regulated by the state board of pharmacy, and this may not be permitted. Providing a full prescription is a significant patient satisfier and may also increase clinic income. Use of lower-cost or generic prescriptions can also improve patient satisfaction and decrease patient costs. In addition, using generics or specific formulary drugs reduces phone calls from pharmacies requiring changes in medications—often from nonformulary medication to formulary medication based on panels of specific insurance carriers, Medicare, and Medicaid. (Please see Appendix B: Supply Inventory List.)

IV fluids and medications are used to treat cellulitis, gastroenteritis, and more serious infections. These interventions can improve and increase clinic charges but decrease room turnover time. They also reduce the number of patients who need to be transferred to a hospital ED. Hospital-affiliated urgent care facilities can provide a relief valve for the ED by performing these services.

Key Takeaway

Location is critical to the success of urgent care centers, including adequate signage, parking, and space based on volume. The decision to lease versus purchase is based on available capital and current market conditions. This varies considerably between a hospital-run facility and an independent, physician-run clinic. Architectural expertise and consultation should be sought for internal design to ensure that local codes are followed and work flow is maximized. Urgent care centers are often required to follow local and state codes for the size of rooms and number of restrooms, among other items. In addition, the site must be cosmetically appealing for patients and family, with an adequate waiting room.

Inventory control and appropriate patient charges are also crucial to avoid lost clinic income. Many venders provide dispensing machines for patient-specific dispensing and charging that can often improve patient safety with allergy or interaction alerts while preventing lost charges quickly exceeding the costs of the equipment. Providing advanced care (e.g., IV fluids) is a management decision, but it can improve per-patient revenue and satisfaction. Remembering to use formulary and generic medications also reduces patient costs, improves patient satisfactions, and reduces staff work by eliminating phone calls from pharmacies.

REFERENCES

1. Huddy, J. 2006. Emergency Department Design: A Practical Guide to Planning for the Future. American College of Emergency Physicians, Dallas, TX.

2. Pash, P. 2008. Failing to Plan or Planning to Fail? Designing a Clinic for Success. J Urgent Care Med. December 2008:34-37.

Billing, Coding, Collections

Patient care volume is critical to urgent care center success, and revenue from this volume is vital in supporting operations and growth. Management must understand the unique aspects of participation with a payer, credentialing, and billing processes. Appropriate documentation and coding will result in solid collections practices that support the finances of the clinic. Documentation and charge capture are both crucial elements to successfully optimize revenue. Billing companies can assist facilities in all of these processes to help maximize reimbursement. The following are key questions owners of urgent care centers should ask regarding billing and collections:

- What is important about timing of a clinic opening and credentialing for specific insurance products?

- What managed care programs should I participate with?

- Should I participate in Medicare? Medicaid?

- How do urgent care centers optimize revenue?

Should we utilize an outside billing company?

- What important aspects of registration apply to insurance and reimbursement?

Insurance Participation Strategies

The lifeblood of all urgent care clinics is volume, and obtaining that volume includes being a preferred provider of managed care organizations (MCO). Depending on the market, there are usually different high-penetration carriers. Delays in either contracting or credentialing with MCOs can significantly impact the finances of your organization. Medicare participation is advised, and Medicaid may be required for hospital-affiliated urgent care sites. Cash collections can enable visits from specific self-pay populations and be used for patients who are insured with a nonparticipating insurance program. Credentialing providers with Medicare and MCOs requires special consideration. Carriers may offer reimbursement as a flat fee or a percentage of Medicare or based on a fee schedule, which is less common.

Understanding basic financial planning, cash flow, and the costs of your clinic is crucial to solid performance. It is important to develop and understand your financial plan, including the costs to run the clinic and the minimum amount of collections required to break even. Knowing the costs of care will allow you to decide if you are able to sign contracts with a global fee, open your doors to the Medicaid population, and treat self-pay patients. By developing a lower cost structure accompanied by solid efficiency (treating adequate volume), your clinic can survive even major economic challenges.

Urgent care owners and administrators should understand that they fund the costs of care—staff, equipment, and facility costs—until reimbursement is received from the insurance company or other payer. This delay in payment can range from 30–90 days and sometimes even longer. Understanding that you are initially funding the cost of care is especially true during the startup phase, when providers must be enrolled into Medicare and Medicaid programs. Payment will not be issued until enrollment in these government programs is complete, which can take several months. You should list in the registration area, on websites, and other communication materials what insurance the facility participates with. In addition, careful consideration should occur before accepting government programs, especially Medicaid.

PUBLICALLY POSTING POLICIES

Your payment and collection policy should be very visible at registration. In addition, posting of a fee schedule for the costs of routine visits and testing may be a positive marketing tool.

Urgent care centers routinely participate in Medicare; however, you should conduct an analysis to verify Medicaid reimbursement and determine the potential patient population the urgent care center may serve from this payer. The following strategies should be considered when approaching other payers:

1. Compare the urgent care center costs to those of local emergency department (ED) visits. This strategy highlights the cost-effectiveness of the urgent care center and the heightened patient satisfaction usually derived from urgent care center visits as compared to ED visits.

2.   Focus on employer groups. Often, the services offered through the urgent care center can be tailored for employer groups in a manner that ensures prompt turnaround and convenient billing. This can result in heightened patient satisfaction, which, in turn, will be seen as significant enhancements to employer groups. Further, this approach allows for the development of a relationship for preemployment exams or testing, routine or annual testing for employees, and occupational medical needs as they arise for the employer group.

3.   Forecasting and modeling volume discounts. In exchange for higher volumes of beneficiaries, the urgent care center may be willing to offer discounts from their normal fees. This can be done with employer groups, and we certainly recommend having employer groups advocate these discounts to their carriers once a solid relationship has been developed or is being developed.

Determining Which Payers to Work With

Managed care plans are intent on reducing inappropriate and costly ED visits. They do this by enforcing higher copays for ED services, directing patients away from the ED via telephone triage programs by offering select participating urgent care sites as an alternative, and using the Internet to direct patients away from the ED. You can capitalize on this opportunity by participating with the major carrier(s) in your area to become a preferred provider of urgent care services. This is accomplished by contacting the provider relations and enrollment department of the specific MCOs.

The major insurance carriers include Blue Cross (Anthem, etc.), United Health Care, Cigna, Humana, Aetna, Kaiser, and the government (Medicare and Medicaid). Governmental coverage approaches more than 50% in some markets. You can determine the dominant players in specific geographic markets through the state insurance commission or by contacting the local healthcare system. There may also be a local health plan sponsored by the health system, an independent practice association/organization, or physician-hospital organization. You must be able to get MCO contracts to survive; it is difficult, and often impossible, to survive on cash collection only. Contracting with the above-mentioned groups can help boost volume for your site.

Hospital-owned or -affiliated urgent care facilities may have a contract group providing services. In this situation, typically the provider group (physician, nurse practitioner, and physician assistant) will bill separately from the hospital, which makes it difficult to develop global fees and sign global fee contracts.

Billing can occur by facility or by a specific provider. Our experience is greater with specific provider enrollment. Understanding the process and time requirements of enrolling specific providers or a facility is essential when determining which payers to contract with. For example, with Medicare, each provider must obtain a Medicare provider identification number (PIN) and provider transaction access number (PTAN). You can apply only 30 days prior to opening, but the process can take many months to complete. Medicare does allow some retroactive payment of claims, but there is a time limit, and many other carriers do not allow retroactive payments. You should consider collecting cash payments in the amount of a copay for other insurance until you are able to bill the carrier directly. Completing the financial credentialing paperwork can be an arduous task, and negotiating a managed care contract can also be difficult.

Contract Negotiations

The MCO process starts with negotiating and signing a contract, followed by credentialing and activation of the provider or clinic. You do not get paid for services until you have been activated by the carrier. Once you have agreed to a managed care contract, all your providers will need to be enrolled for payment. Completing the financial credentialing paperwork the correct way the first time is essential. This is an area in which billing companies can be of assistance. The credentialing process for providers can take 180 days or more, and being adversarial with the carrier will only make the process even longer (you may even be ignored). Delays usually occur, and it is vital that someone stays on top of the credentialing process to ensure that all of the providers are enrolled, if you are not simply enrolling the facility and billing under a facility contract. Even with facility contracts, the providers will require some credentialing.

Critical components of MCO contracts include submission of clean claims, issues regarding denials, the length of the contract, and the ability to terminate the contract. It is crucial that you—and your legal counsel or billing company—read all of the fine print in the managed care contract.

Clean claims indicate those cases where the bill is paid without any chart review—your money comes back faster, reducing accounts receivable (AR) days. The MCO may have a very stringent policy that delays the payment of claims for "review purposes," meaning they hold your money as an interest-free loan for longer periods of time, resulting in higher AR days for your clinic. You should also understand the denial process and what steps can be taken to challenge this process and appeal the case. Some MCOs will deny payment due to lack of prior authorization for the visit. You should attempt to eliminate these types of clauses during the initial negotiations or, if present, ensure that the registration staff obtains preauthorization for all applicable patients.

Contracts are often negotiated for multiyear implementation, so it is important that you ensure that an annual escalator clause of 2%–3% is in place to cover the costs of inflation and other increased costs of doing the business. Finally, you should know the length of contracts and reasons for termination. If a large MCO simply terminates your agreement, this may drop your volume by 50%, resulting in potential insolvency.

The structure of the urgent care center, to a large extent, will determine whether a new tax identification number or the organization's existing tax identification will be used for billing purposes. For instance, if a hospital is developing an urgent care center, either independently or in a partnership with physicians, it will most likely use an existing tax identification number. This becomes important, because existing payer contracts will need to be honored for billing the urgent care center services. Many payer contracts exclude urgent care center payment or limit urgent care center payment after a significant copayment. It will be important to understand the payment ramifications for the urgent care center when making a decision on the center's structure and which tax identification number will be used.

,lling for Services

There seems to be some question about what services urgent care practices can bill for, what they actually do bill for, and what they can actually get reimbursed for. In reality, the nature of urgent care medicine coding and billing is fairly straightforward.

When comparing urgent care codes to ED evaluation and management (E/M) codes 99281 and 99285, critical care codes 99291 and 99292, and hospital observation codes 99218, 99220, 99234, and 99236, urgent care centers use the more traditional new and established patient CPT codes, such as 99201 and 99205. Additionally, many urgent care centers generate only one bill, so all procedures, laboratory, radiology, and supplies are combined on the single bill. With hospital-affiliated programs, the physician (and MLP) are subcontracted, billing may be done through the provider (not utilizing the common charge sheet) and facility separately. Some MCOs only reimburse the professional component disallowing any facility fee. Obviously, the facility charges for supplies and testing, but may be denied a specific additional facility fee. Having an emphasis on proper documentation and charge capture is important to successfully optimize revenue.

When working with your urgent care services team, there should be a shared, coordinated, and highly collaborative focus on accurate and timely documentation. Further, it is essential that the charge sheet used by the clinical services team is comprehensive in identifying the level of care, all laboratory services, all radiographic services, all supplies, and all procedures performed. This charge sheet will be the source document for driving the CPT code established and used.

In our experience, urgent care centers generate an average charge per visit of $300.00. Depending on payer contracts and third-party participation, it is common for the urgent care center to collect between 40% and 50% of their visit charge. Strategies to improve collections include:

- Using electronic registration

- Using real-time charge entry with the electronic registration

- Billing electronically for all payers, if possible

- Developing protocols for real-time insurance verification and portion of bills paid by insurance

- Collecting deductibles and copays at the time services are rendered

- Printing demand bills for the patient/guarantor as they complete their visit

Use of midlevel providers

Midlevel providers (MLP), such as physician assistants or nurse practitioners, are effective service providers in an urgent care center, but some insurance carriers will require that patients be evaluated by a physician. In our experience, this is more the exception than the rule. More commonly, we find that a physician needs to be available for consultation and supervision of the MLP. These requirements are determined by state law but may be more stringent with an MCO contract.

The MLP is effective for handling less-acute patients and providing additional service capacity. Peak times for additional staffing include midafternoon, when school gets out, and after 5:00 p.m. or 5:30 p.m., when work gets out. You should ensure that you are paid for the services provided by the MLP and avoid any contract clause that disallows this or makes the process arduous. From a billing and coding perspective, the services rendered by the MLP are often attested by and billed under the supervising physician's signature. However, many carriers allow billing under the MLP (review contractual requirements before billing submission). From a coding and billing perspective, the documentation must be comprehensive and the chargemaster forms complete, and both must be legible. Most billing will be done under the center's tax identification number and use the physician's signature and attestation in order to generate the claim.

Patient registration

Correct patient information and insurance documentation are fundamental to establishing collection policies that are successful. Accurate patient information reduces claims denials for incorrect patient name, address, and member number. If claims are delayed, this also hampers payment for services. For example, invoices are often returned due to incorrect addresses. If the patient has visited the center in the past, it is critical to closely verify that the information is still correct. Scanning devices are available for both license and insurance cards, reducing the need for copying and improving efficiency.

In addition, insurance verification can help reduce lost revenue even with a specific member card, and further verification should be done with Medicaid patients. Often, this can be accomplished through Internet communication. The verification should also include details of copays for urgent care sites and the amount of deductibles.

Finally, we have two sites in New York that allow patients to register via the Internet or phone call. This reduces waiting time and may enhance staff efficiency.

Copays

Copay collections are an important component of payment. Copays in urgent care sites are frequently lower than those in EDs (approximately $50–$200) but higher than those in private physician offices ($20–$50). Collection at the time of service by cash, credit card, or check improves collection. Failure to collect copays and verify insurance may result in the need to directly bill the patient resulting in AR delays and lost revenue.

Facilities should consider collecting a component of the bill for those patients who have an insurance deductible (especially with high deductible policies). These payments act as a deposit and are very helpful in the first half of the year, when deductibles are often unmet. Collecting deductibles is critical with patients who are maintaining health savings accounts, because the cost of the visit is often lower than the high-deductible policy. Patients or legal guardians should be provided with billing policies and procedures during the registration process. They should also be required to sign statements for financial responsibility if the claim is denied by the carrier.

Documentation and coding

Based on Medicare requirements, specific components are necessary to be recorded on the chart to qualify for reimbursement at specific acuity levels. The lack of documentation can result in decreased reimbursement. This is especially true regarding urgent care centers and new patients, because any new encounter requires documentation of a patient's past medical, family, and social history. New patients without this specific documentation will be placed in lower levels of coding and reimbursement. Urgent care should be coded as such and not as care provided at a physician office or practice. In addition, afterhours, weekend, and holiday charges are allowable. The urgent care clinics often focus on episodic, clinical events that involve injury or illness. Providing routine primary care services through your site may impair your ability to bill as an urgent care center.

Global fees can be negotiated but should be above your per-patient costs, plus additional profit. These fees are beneficial when you care for low-acuity visits, such as those conditions often treated in a retail clinic. You may be offered a flat rate, but you need to understand that you will be paid the same for treating the sore throat requiring only a prescription, sewing up a laceration that takes an hour, and treating a dehydrated patient over several hours with IV fluids. Developing carve-outs with MCOs for higher-acuity cases, such as laceration repairs, incision and drainage of abscesses, and cases requiring testing (i.e., labs and x-rays), is essential to urgent care clinic viability. Your competition may negotiate a poor contract with discounted rates. These practices often result in lower margins and may end in clinic failure—know your costs of care and do not accept lower payment.

In addition, billing should occur under point of service 20 (urgent care center) rather than 11 (physician office). The majority of your visits should be unscheduled, episodic, and for acute illness or injury.

Billing companies

Experienced billing companies can help urgent care sites immensely with many of the above-mentioned issues. For example, they can provide expertise in reviewing and negotiating managed care contracts, credentialing with MCOs, credentialing with Medicare and Medicaid, providing electronic claims submission to reduce the time it takes to receive payment, and decreasing AR days and help manage claims denials.

They can also provide feedback on provider documentation offering potential opportunities for improvement. Vast educational resources are available from these companies. However, you should consider only those companies with experience and expertise in urgent care and emergency medicine that bill more than 500,000 claims per year and can file the majority of claims electronically.

Costs for a quality company can range from 8%–9% of billed charges. There are many companies that are less expensive; however, you get what you pay for, and you cannot afford to have a bad billing company. Poorly performing billing companies can destroy your finances, prolong AR, and result in many patient complaints that can cause a loss of business.

Key Takeaway

You should use great caution in contract negotiations with MCOs and only accept what you can afford. Often, the MCO will negotiate very aggressively and provide a take-it-or-leave-it option. Again, we cannot emphasize enough the importance of knowing your costs before signing a bad agreement, along with knowing the expected volume from the MCO. Your competitor down the street may not be as business savvy and may accept a very low rate. Still, you should not accept what you cannot afford, and patience may bring the business to you anyway after your competition fails. It is critical to complete provider credentialing quickly and abide by all the requirements in the MCO contract to avoid receiving the following statement: "No credentialing, no preauthorization, no payment, and denied as out of network or failure to obtain preauthorization."

Coding and documentation are also important in order to bill for the appropriate level of services provided. Finally, experienced billing companies can provide significant assistance in managed care notifications, practice assessment, documentation assistance, and management of clinic finances (e.g., accounts receivable, aging accounts, and bad debt).

6

Human Resources and Staffing

A key component to the success of an urgent care center is the personnel providing patient care, also known as the urgent care team. After the initial costs for
the clinic startup, staffing expenses are usually the greatest component of a
center's budget. It is imperative to hire staff members with the right attributes,
such as the necessary skill set, a positive personality, and flexibility. You also
need to understand the basics of certification, licensure, and who can provide
specific levels of care. For example, a nurse practitioner may repair lacerations,
whereas medical assistants cannot. Likewise, intravenous (IV) administration of
conscious sedation medication may need to be done by a registered nurse. It's the
job of physicians and clinic managers to know the laws and regulations regarding who can perform venipuncture, lab tests, and other procedures.[1] The following are common staffing questions.

- How many staff members do I need to run my clinic?

- Can a nurse practitioner practice alone in the clinic?

- What are the optimal hours of operation?

- What will my wage costs be?

STAFFING DEFINITIONS AND DESCRIPTIONS OF PERSONNEL

Certification: Typically provided by a professional organization attesting that an individual has successfully completed requirements of a course and, often, passed a written exam and/or practical skills test (e.g., advanced cardiac life support certification).

Licensure: The legal permission granted by states or municipalities to perform specific acts.

Licensed practical nurse/licensed vocational nurse (LVN): These clinicians typically undergo at least a one-year training program through vocational schools or community colleges, with some programs extending to a two-year associate's degree. Level-of-care limitations may not allow medication dose titration, provision of the first dose of IV antibiotics, and IV push medications. These limitations are dependent on the regulations of the facility and municipality (state). Teaching programs focus on clinical skills as opposed to medical theory and in-depth pathophysiology of disease that are taught to registered nurses and bachelor's-level nursing programs. The terminology licensed vocational nurse is more often utilized in the states of Texas and California. The titles are essentially interchangeable, and each nurse must work under the direct supervision of a registered nurse or a physician.

Medical assistant: These providers have varied skill levels, training, and experience. State guidelines may be in place determining the level of practice that these clinicians can perform. They often do a variety of clerical, administrative, and clinical tasks. At a minimum, they have the ability to take vital signs and set up equipment for procedures and can apply simple dressings without medication application. Training programs include certificates and associate's degrees from vocational and technical schools and community colleges, with varied length of training, from six months to two years, with professional organization registration or certification.

Registered nurse (RN): RNs may have completed a two-year associate's degree registered nurse program or a four-year Bachelor of Science degree in nursing (BSN),

STAFFING DEFINITIONS AND DESCRIPTIONS OF PERSONNEL (CONT.)

and need to maintain a state license with the ability to provide all levels of nursing care. The BSN programs provide greater detail and education into the pathophysiology of disease along with management aspects of patient care and nursing administration.

Nurse practitioner (NP): NPs have completed a four-year bachelor's degree along with two or more years of nurse practitioner training at the master's or doctoral level and state licensing through the board of nursing. They have prescriptive authority for most medications and greater independent practice ability compared to physician assistants. NPs perform the same types of urgent care procedures that physician assistants can perform, including laceration repair, abscess drainage, nasal procedures, etc. Their ability to function independently is based on each state's specific nurse practice act.[2]

Physician assistant (PA): PAs have completed a four-year bachelor's degree, an additional 1–2 years of PA school at the master's level, and licensing through the state medical board. Some older programs take less than four years to complete, and some four-year programs are bachelor's degree only that may result in limitations with billing and Medicare. PAs have prescriptive authority for most medications and collaborative practice agreements that often require supervision from an on-site physician. PAs cannot practice independently, requiring employment or contracting with a supervising physician in order to practice.[3] Still, PAs can perform many of the same types of urgent care procedures as NPs, including laceration repair, abscess drainage, nasal procedures, fracture care, etc.

They provide care and practice under the license of a physician with delegated authority from that physician. Often, states, facilities, or malpractice insurance carriers will require documents describing the specific practices the PA is allowed to do by the physician under a written delegated authority agreement. Several states allow independent practice, with specific information being available along with requirements through each state's medical board. Although licensing is not required, providers without a

STAFFING DEFINITIONS AND DESCRIPTIONS OF PERSONNEL (CONT.)

license may have difficulty with credentialing and billing for services. It is critical to understand a state's requirements for oversight and independent practice restrictions. In addition, Medicare and other insurance carriers may reimburse differently for mid-level providers (MLP). Failure to follow specified billing guidelines for MLPs may result in allegations of fraudulent billing practices.

Practice manager, office manager, or operation director: This person may or may not have a clinical background, but there is a major benefit in having knowledge of medical office flow, ancillary service use, provider staffing, managed care negotiations, supply and inventory control, and facility budgeting. The ideal person for this position in a hospital-affiliated or owned site would be a BSN nurse with significant management experience. This position is recommended for sites with six or more beds.

Family physician: These physicians have completed medical school along with training of three or more years of family practice residency. Programs focus on inpatient and outpatient care with education on care for all ages, wellness, and care for chronic diseases.

Internal medicine physician: These physicians have completed medical school along with training of three or more years of internal medicine residency. Programs focus on inpatient and outpatient care, with education focused toward adults, wellness, and care for chronic disease, including hypertension and diabetes. Education, training, and clinical experience in pediatrics is often very limited.

Emergency physician: These physicians have completed medical school along with training of three or more years of emergency medicine residency. Programs focus on critical care, resuscitation, procedural skills, and trauma for all ages. In addition, education includes all aspects of medical and surgical illness and disease. The focus is dedicated on the treatment of episodic illness and injuries.

Hiring the Right People

The lifeblood of every clinic is the staff members who care for each patient. Not only is staffing the largest component of a clinic's budget, it has a major impact on patient satisfaction, which results in return business. When starting a clinic, employee interviews are critical to build your A team, because you want to field your best team every day. Most administrators know what attributes make up an A-team employee, but certain personality characteristics are vital. According to the book *Leadership for Great Customer Service: Satisfied Patient, Satisfied Employees*, these personality characteristics include the following mannerisms: positive, proactive, confident, competent, compassionate, communicator, team player, and trustworthy. These people do what it takes to get the job done and maintain a sense of humor in the process.[4] In the interview process, you can discover these traits and specifically ask the interviewee about opinions regarding patient satisfaction and customer service. Negative responses should send up red flags. Urgent care centers are much more prone to losing business from poor service than other healthcare facilities. Not only should this evaluation be part of the hiring process, but ongoing training on customer service is critical for all staff members.

Staffing Requirements

The ideal staffing of an urgent care clinic is highly dependent on the intended level of clinical care, budget available, and provider staff practices based on state/jurisdiction allowance. There are very cost-effective models that can be implemented with graduated skill levels of providers. As has been discussed previously, all facilities must abide by state regulation regarding practices that specifically pertain to medical assistant versus LVN, LVN versus RN, and MLP versus physician. If independent practice by a nonphysician is considered, the site will need to determine the appropriate model, with nurse practitioner or physician assistant.

Volume projections

One crucial element of staffing appropriately is having a correct projection of volume and clinic productivity. Many office practices tout that caring for four to six patients per hour is easily accomplished, but we find that this number far exceeds what can be safely accomplished in an urgent care clinic. An office practice cares for a known population of established patients that makes visits much shorter. But many urgent care sites have a majority of new patient visits, especially during the first two years of operation. The new-patient visits and the documentation requirements limit the upside potential per provider from a low of two patients per hour to a high of four patients per hour. This productivity is heavily dependent on the support staff and nursing to be efficient with flow. Finally, the specialty and background of the physician play a significant role and are important in relation to costs, speed, and test utilization with patient care.

Work flow patterns

Patient flow is directly dependent on the acuity level of the urgent care patient and the test utilization habits of the provider involved. It is important to realize that physician practice patterns vary. Previous training suggests different points of focus by specialty. Family physicians and internists are traditionally outpatient focused and likely view the patient's complaint with the mind-set of, "What is the most likely diagnosis of the patient with this complaint in an office environment?" Emergency physicians are trained to start with the worst-case scenario, so their thought process starts with, "What will kill my patient with this complaint in any environment?" and then they work backward.

For example, the family physician may assess the patient with leg pain and feel it is muscular in nature, whereas the emergency physician may see the same patient and consider that the patient needs to have a Doppler exam to rule out a deep vein thrombosis. Neither approach is incorrect, but the scenario provides a frame of reference. In addition, some physicians can be described as high-test utilizers with high risk aversion (I don't want to miss anything or I will be sued) or low-test utilizers (the odds are that this patient does not have something bad and doesn't need that extra test). There is no right or wrong practice method; they are simply different. From an urgent care center standpoint, a high-test utilizer will increase costs of care and turnaround time. They may, however, detect a diagnosis that the low-test utilizer would not. It is difficult to retrain physicians that have a history of high-test utilization.

The majority of urgent care clinics are staffed by family physicians and emergency physicians, followed by internists, pediatricians, and other specialties.[5] We have found that family physicians and intermediate- to low-test utilizer emergency physicians work best in the urgent care environment. They have solid flow and turnaround times, with ratios of 2.2–3.5 patients per hour, whereas the high-test utilizer will often have productivity of less than two patients per hour. The difference between the two practice patterns significantly affects flow and patient satisfaction. Internists fall closer to the family physician practice pattern. For the internist, there may be clinical areas of weakness that were minimally covered in previous training, including caring for pediatric patients, minor trauma, and wound care. Similarly, pediatricians may have difficulty with adult evaluation, trauma, and wound care.

Employment models

The majority of the staff members at urgent care centers are employees of the site or organization that owns the site. The providers, including physicians, nurse practitioners, and physician assistants, have various relationships to the site depending on the desires of the organization and nonprofit versus for-profit status. The relationship includes employment of the healthcare providers, with each being on a salary with a benefits structure; the second option includes a joint venture structure where the providers participate in the success of the operation by sharing in the profits or losses; and the third option is a contracted entity operating either on an independent fee-for-service basis or hourly charge to the facility.

We are the most familiar with the third component, as we contract for services at hospital-owned facilities. In this situation, the group is formed under a limited liability partnership (LLP) and contracts with the healthcare system. Patients are billed separately for professional services, resulting in a facility charge (charges for facility testing and supplies) and professional fee. Depending on the situation, e.g., site collections, level of staffing, and payer mix, the physician group or LLP may operate without financial assistance from the clinic or may require assistance in the form of a subsidy to make up for costs over accounts receivable.

Staffing Hours

Urgent care hours of operation vary by the site and the desire to draw volume. Afterhours and weekend openings are vital to draw volume from patients who are unable to make routine office appointments with private physicians. In addition, families often are unable to make appointments due to weekday work schedules. In order to maximize volume, planning the hours of operation can be quite challenging and have a direct impact on costs. Typical shifts are scheduled at 8, 10, and 12 hours, with combinations to maximize efficiency and staff desires.

Overtime

Most state and federal guidelines require payment of overtime for greater than 80 hours of work in a two-week period. Many organizations and physician offices attempt to avoid the issue by not paying appropriate overtime, but there are significant sanctions and fines if the site is found to be noncompliant with overtime guidelines.

Opening the facility doors at 9 a.m. and closing at 9 p.m. maximizes hours, but the 12-hour shift causes issues with automatic overtime unless adequate numbers of providers are hired. Hiring two MLPs with a third part-time MLP reduces the effect of the overtime issue and provides for staffing flexibility in regard to illness and vacations. The part-time MLP typically would not receive benefits, which is also a cost savings.

In our system, the most cost-effective model is 12 hours. The most cost-effective staffing for MLP supplementation to physician coverage would be 10- or 12-hour shifts, rotating three shifts on and four shifts off, then four shifts on and three shifts of. This pattern reduces overtime but also provides longer shifts that are appealing to the providers. Most providers prefer longer shifts to reduce the number of shifts they are required to work per month.

Hours of operation

Most urgent care sites remain open until 8 p.m., with some extending hours until 11 p.m. or midnight. Weekend hours should be similar if the volume can be sustained for the extended hours of operation. Some sites close on Sundays, but all of our sites are open seven days per week. We also have coverage on all holidays, with a minimum of eight clinic hours.

Closing policy

The last hour of operation is a significant issue in facilities not operating 24 hours per day. Each urgent care center needs to develop specific closing policies. For example, all of our sites usually close the doors and complete care a minimum of 30 minutes after closing time. Your community will know the closing time and people will rush in at the last minute. You must develop a policy of when to close the door and refer the patients to another site for care. One consideration is to have the closing time listed 30 minutes prior to actual closing by stating no patient will be registered after 8:30 p.m. with a 9 p.m. closure.

Staffing Based on Clinic Model

The purpose of the clinic will play a large role in determining what types of providers and the number of staff required at your urgent care clinic.

DETERMINING THE HOURS OF OPERATION

We were faced with a staffing dilemma at one urgent care site where a nearby hospital was closing. Our plan was to reopen the previous ED as an urgent care center. The community had an ED that was open 24 hours per day, seven days per week prior to the hospital closure. The economics of the area were a significant negative issue, but the neighboring community had an ED that was only 15 minutes away.

Our discussion was whether we should have 12 hours versus 16 hours of operation. We made the decision to provide 12 hours of coverage; this required only one staffing shift, keeping the cost of personnel lower. The community has adjusted to these hours of operation, with a volume of 80 patients per day within the 12-hour period. Sites that have a better revenue source (payer mix) should consider a cost-benefit analysis with additional staffing hours with the option of up to 18 hours of service. Urgent care centers are typically cost-effective, because they are open only during peak volumes hours and do not incur the cost of a 24/7 operation. Finally, you need a pool of qualified nurses (and other staff members) to hire. If there is a lack of qualified personnel to recruit in the area, it may also impact or reduce the hours of operation.

Cash clinic

The purpose of the cash clinic is essentially to provide care at a very low cost and charge based on the patient's ability to pay. The focus is a lower level acuity, with episodic illness and minor injury care for uninsured or underinsured patients. As these sites are smaller (three to five beds), they require only a single provider. Because of the low acuity of conditions being treated, often you can staff these sites with an NP that would substantially reduce costs.

Medical oversight can be immediately available by phone, but with some technical innovation, real-time telemedical consultations could be also provided but would likely incur a cost. Additional staffing requirements include a receptionist, RN, and MA for a census of about 35–45 patients per day. This model can be adjusted up or down based on higher or lower volumes. Rates for care (exclusive of any testing costs) may range between $35–$50 per visit.

Retail clinic

Most retail clinics are staffed with nurse practitioners. Regulatory changes, including the approval of prescriptive authority and mandatory reimbursement for NP and PA services, influenced the increased ability for NPs and PAs to practice independently.[6] Based on the current independent practice ability of these clinicians, many retail clinics depend on them to staff this urgent care model.

The provider is the receptionist, registration person, and nurse; administers medications and injections; and provides discharge education to the patient. These sites are located within existing retail establishments and often have minimum space of one to two rooms. With the very limited nature of the illnesses cared for, technology efficiencies utilized, and lower overhead costs, retail clinics are becoming a significant provider of episodic care. As was discussed in Chapter 1, these sites, along with cash clinics and standard urgent care, facilities can provide treatment for patients who are medically screened out of the ED to a clinic setting.

Full-service urgent care clinic

From a human resources standpoint, full service urgent care sites require significantly greater manpower and seem to represent the majority of current urgent care sites. Support personnel often include a minimum of one registration clerk, one MA, an RN and an LVN, a physician, and an MLP. Space requirements range from 6–10 beds with 3,000–4,500 square feet.

These sites may include imaging that requires a radiology technologist and some laboratory services requiring a certified laboratory technologist as well. Volume and hours of operation vary, but most sites close before midnight, eliminating the need for more than two staffing shifts. Depending on the hours of operation, each site should easily handle 60–80 patients per day. Larger clinics often require a practice manager, office manager, or administrative designate. This person should ensure that staffing, supplies, marketing, and other critical business elements are accomplished, leading to the success of the clinic. Figure 6.1 provides average salaries as obtained from a career source website that provides some ideas of costs.

FIGURE 6.1

MEDIAN YEARLY INCOME OF MEDICAL STAFF IN THE UNITED STATES

MEDICAL STAFF	ANNUAL	HOURLY	COMMENTS
Receptionist	$25,200	$12.14	
Medical assistant	$28,900	$13.87	
Licensed vocational nurse	$40,400	$19.42	
Registered nurse	$64,700	$31.10	Based on a national average of all registered nurses, rate may be lower for clinic
NP/PA	$80,000+	$35–55/hour	Employed, based on experience, data from ECI
Physician	$150,000+	$80–120/hour	Depending on employment or contractor relationship

Source: www.careeronestop.org

Chapter 6

REFERENCES

1. Lewis, M., Tamparo, C. 2007. Medical Law, Ethics, and Bioethics for Ambulatory Care, 6th ed. F.A Davis Company, Philadelphia, PA.

2. Curren, J. 2007. Nurse Practitioners and Physician Assistants: Do You Know the Difference. MedSurg Nursing. 16(6):404–407.

3. Perry, J. 2009. The Rise and Impact of Nurse Practitioners and Physician Assistants on Their Own and Cross-Occupation Incomes. Contemporary Economic Policy. 27(4):491–511.

4. Mayer, T., Cates, R. 2004. Leadership for Great Customer Service: Satisfied Patient, Satisfied Employees. Health Administrative Press, Chicago, IL.

5. Weinick, R., Bristol, S., DesRoches, C. 2009 Urgent care centers in the U.S.: Findings from a national survey. BMC Health Services Research. 9(Special section):1–8.

6. Curren, J. 2007. Nurse Practitioners and Physician Assistants: Do You Know the Difference. MedSurg Nursing. 16(6):404–407.

7

Ancillary Testing: Laboratory and Radiology Services

Ancillary services, including laboratory and radiographic testing, are available in the majority of urgent care centers. Laboratory services can vary from a simple bedside glucose or pregnancy test to full-service lab capabilities. Radiographic testing may be limited to plain musculoskeletal films or can include a complete imaging facility including plain x-rays, CT scans, ultrasounds, mammography, and bone density scanning.

The presence of both laboratory and radiology services can increase patient volume for urgent care sites. At our centers, the presence of each of these services (e.g., imaging center, laboratory, or a draw station) helps to augment the volume of the other ancillary site. For example, an outpatient imaging center will be used by community physicians, and patient traffic to that imaging center provides free marketing to an adjacent urgent care clinic. An outpatient laboratory (or even a draw station) can provide similar patient traffic and marketing opportunities for urgent care clinics. The following are four common questions regarding laboratory and radiology services that urgent care administrators should ask:

- Should the clinic provide laboratory testing, i.e., waive or nonwaive testing?

- What costs are involved in a Clinical Laboratory Improvement Amendment (CLIA)–certified laboratory?

- Should the clinic provide radiology exams?

- What studies are available in a freestanding imaging center?

Our urgent care center experience in New York demonstrates provider test utilization as a percentage of volume between 18% and 20% for radiologic exams, 17% and 22% for laboratory tests (mostly waive tests), and about 4% for both. These urgent care sites are hospital affiliated and have full-service imaging centers (e.g., computerized radiography [CR] for musculoskeletal films, CT, mammography, ultrasound, bone density, and limited MRI) as well as waive testing labs (e.g., H/H, pregnancy, strep screen, influenza, monospot, urine dipstick, Chem 8). The waive testing area also includes a draw station for the main hospital laboratory. The majority of radiographic studies ordered at the urgent care site are plain musculoskeletal radiographs followed by CT scanning. The urgent care center's radiographic and laboratory services are also extensively used by community physicians.

ANCILLARY DEFINITIONS

Carve-out: A term utilized with the billing process to describe removal or separation of a medical test or procedure from a contract and paid under a different arrangement.

CLIA: The Clinical Laboratory Improvement Amendment sets minimum standards for labs to follow.

Computed radiography (CR): CR uses phosphor material plates in cassettes. After exposed to x-rays, the cassettes are scanned by lasers in a digitizer producing the image.

Computed tomography (CT): Axial cuts (cross-sectional) of the body produced by ionizing radiation. The series of sectional, planar images may be reformatted using computer technology to provide a multidimensional picture.

DICOM: Digital imaging and communication in medicine format is a standard storage process for digital radiographic images.

Direct radiography (DR): The detector is directly exposed to x-rays, which eliminates the need for cassettes and a digitizer.[1]

Digital radiography: The capture or conversion of radiographic images in a digital format.

General radiology: Images of the skull, chest, abdomen, spine, and extremities produced by the basic radiographic process.

Mammography: A modality utilizing ionic x-ray imaging for breast examinations.

Magnetic resonance imaging (MRI): This test uses a magnetic field and pulses of radio wave energy to make pictures of organs and structures inside the body.

Picture Archiving and Communication System (PACS): The digital capture, transfer, and storage of diagnostic images. It consists of a networked computer system including a

---

ANCILLARY DEFINITIONS (CONT.)

server with stations providing the ability for viewing, manipulation, and interpretation of images.

Ultrasound: High-frequency sound waves are utilized to determine the size and shape of internal organs based on the differential rates of reflection. Real-time images may include coloration evaluating arterial and venous flow.

Waive testing: Lab tests that are considered simple to perform with very low potential for error (e.g., bedside glucose testing and urine pregnancy tests) and do not require annual laboratory inspection but require a CLIA certificate of waiver for waive testing.

Determining What Laboratory Services to Provide

As you are contemplating the degree to which you want to provide laboratory services in your urgent care site, you should consider the following.

- Your clinicians will routinely need access to lab testing for flu, strep, mono, pregnancy, and urine tests.

- Having point-of-care testing can improve your site's efficiency, speed, and cost-effectiveness.

- According to the National Association for Ambulatory Care (NAFAC), 98% of all urgent care centers have a CLIA level II laboratory for routine blood test and other diagnostic procedures. To be a waived test under CLIA, the test must be easy to interpret with little potential for error and

---

able to be performed by most staff with the appropriate training. The facility is required to have a CLIA certificate of waiver, as well.

Maintaining laboratory services in urgent care sites requires appropriate certification, ongoing monitoring, and inspection by professional, state, and other regulatory agencies. Lab requirements vary by state and type of urgent care ownership model—hospital-affiliated facilities, for example, usually having greater requirements than private offices. In addition, staffing requirements vary depending on the level of laboratory services offered. For example, small CLIA-waived labs may require a technician or nurse to perform testing, whereas larger labs may require a medical technologist with at least a four-year college degree to perform testing and oversight along with a medical director.

Cost considerations

The costs of tabletop testing units have been dramatically reduced in recent years, including processors/analyzers for hematology (CBC with automated differential) and chemistry testing (providing basic and comprehensive metabolic profiles). Some of the benefits of having these types of in-house testing include quicker results, rapid supplemental information to provide a patient's diagnosis, reduced amount of time spent tracking results for tests that are sent out to labs and follow-up calls to patients, and a decreased number of lost specimens.[2]

We have found that in-house processors/analyzers could be purchased for well under $100,000 or far cheaper if you purchase quality, refurbished equipment. The additional costs of compliance testing, ongoing certification, materials/reagents, proficiency testing, and staffing higher-trained personnel (e.g., a technician versus technologist) should be added to the instrument costs to determine the true costs of the lab. For example, the average annual salary for a laboratory technician in the United States is $36,500, compared to a laboratory technologist at $56,100, according to *careeronestop.org*. Urgent care centers may be required to staff the higher-paid lab technologist with larger, nonwaive lab programs.

Nonwaive test labs require development of policies and procedures, proficiency testing, and extensive documentation (i.e., training, quality assurance, mainte- nance). To perform nonwaive testing, the clinic requires both certification and accreditation that can be obtained through one of the three agencies below:

1. The Commission on Office and Laboratory Accreditation: Used by smaller labs and physician offices, cheapest alternative (*www.cola.org*)

2. The American College of Pathologists (*www.cap.org*)

3. The Joint Commission (*www.jointcommission.org*)

Investing in new analyzers may reduce costs per test to less than $3 compared with higher costs per waived test at $10–$15, which is dependent on the total number and type of tests conducted, as well as the cost per kit for waived tests. Reimbursement for many lab tests is limited and often is just over $10 per test based on Medicare levels (further information on reimbursement levels can be found at *www.cms.gov/ClinicalLabFeeSched*).

As a simple mathematics formula demonstrates (10 − 3 = \$7 versus 10 − 10 = \$0), the profit potential appears to be far greater for urgent care sites that purchase the "tabletop analyzer" than those using the waive test model. But it is important to perform a cost analysis by estimating the total number of tests that the clinic could perform and estimating the potential income. You then need to subtract the above-described costs when determining profit or loss. As most administrators and physicians are aware, reimbursement for tests also varies by carrier, but it is unlikely that reimbursement will increase. Each state has different requirements that can have a direct impact on cost and reimbursement, as well.

Conversely, CLIA waive testing requires minimal training, oversight, and auditing that results in potentially lower overall costs. The urgent care site is required to have a certificate of waiver for waived testing through one of the above-mentioned agencies at a cost of \$150 every two years. Of 430 urgent care centers audited, 93.3% performed some type of testing, with 87.2% falling under the CLIA waive testing category. Moderate testing complexity occurred in 37% of urgent care sites and full lab certification occurred in 21%.[3]

If your intent is to keep production costs low, such as in a cash clinic model, lab technology should be minimized and waive testing should be strongly considered. In order to make the best use of tabletop analyzers, you should have a significantly higher volume of patients than a typical urgent care site cares for and perform a detailed cost analysis that includes all costs prior to equipment purchase.

Finally, it is imperative for the urgent care center administrator or manager to continuously review the top 10–15 lab tests performed and compare the cost reimbursement for each test to ensure that the cost is not greater than reimbursement. You should also ensure that you are either reimbursed at a high-enough level from all your bundled service agreements with managed care contracts to make up for the costs of ancillary testing, or these lab tests need to be carved out of the bundled service and paid for separately.

One piece of lab equipment to keep in mind that is relatively inexpensive and enables physicians to perform several diagnostic studies is a laboratory microscope. Quality microscopes can be purchased for approximately $1,000. Tests that can be conducted with these types of microscopes are vaginal wet preps (saline and potassium hydroxide), analysis of skin scrapings, review of peripheral blood smears, and urine specimens.

We have found that urgent care clinics with limited lab testing benefit from a reduced number of lab delays and increased throughput. Sites with full-service lab capabilities benefit from increased utilization of laboratory services but often also experience prolonged turnaround times.

At our sites, providers are contractors to the site and there is not a financial incentive to increased test utilization. We believe the more tests practitioners have available, the more they will utilize tests, which can be a two-edged sword. Urgent care sites that lack expanded lab testing capabilities will likely have a higher number of patient transfers to emergency departments (ED) or hospitals to obtain advanced lab tests. Our experience yields an average 2%–3% transfer rate per urgent care site, with half of the patients requiring hospital admission and half requiring additional testing, the most common test being an afterhours ultrasound.

Determining What Radiology Services to Provide

The majority of urgent care centers we are involved with have plain radiography (musculoskeletal) and most also have both CT scanning and ultrasound. R. Weinick's study, "Urgent Care Centers in the U.S.: Findings from a National Survey," found that out of the 430 urgent care center respondents, 14% had CT scanning and 18.6% had ultrasound.[4] Based on our experience, 18%–25% of urgent care patient visits require at least one radiographic study. Yet, one of the greatest challenges for urgent care is the potential need for preauthorization of testing for advanced diagnostic imaging, especially MRI studies. Without preauthorization, reimbursement for the imaging test may be denied. There are many professional consultants who can help you evaluate radiographic equipment before purchase, and they can make recommendations for your facility on topics such as space utilization, purchasing new versus used equipment, and work flow design.

Radiologic services require both significant capital and space. It is critical to understand both the purchase costs of the equipment, equipment options, imaging type, and the maintenance costs. The following questions are a good starting point when determining what level of imaging services to provide.

- What are the benefits and drawback of lease versus purchase options?

- What is the equipment's typical lifespan and its salvage value at the end of its lifespan?

- Does purchasing new or refurbished equipment best fit your needs?

- What level of radiation exposure risk is there from both a patient and staff perspective?

Before opening an imaging center with radiology services, a state certified medical physicist needs to assess the radiation exposure and ensure that the structure has appropriate leading of walls. Without this certification, you will be unable to occupy the site until that requirement has been rectified.

Cost considerations

Imaging equipment can be conventional (film based) or digital (CR or DR). Conventional radiology is the traditional film-based program with equipment that is cheaper for a clinic to purchase. However, an article by T. Hale, "Technology in Urgent Care: Digital or Conventional Imaging?" suggests that this notion of conventional radiology being cheaper may not be correct after you factor in all of the related costs.[5] For example, conventional systems require film, film processors, additional space for the processor, and film storage. Film also requires greater time for processing, and there is sometimes a need to repeat the test when image film quality or views are inadequate.

CR allows image capture on a cassette that is inserted in a digitizer. The image is produced in less than three minutes by a laser scanner and is stored in a DICOM format.[6] DR does not utilize a cassette or digitizer; instead, it has a detector that captures x-ray increasing the speed of image acquisition and improves quality. DR is more expensive than CR, but prices of the former have been falling drastically.

Both types of digital imaging have improved image quality and easier image manipulation compared to conventional radiography. Digital images are also captured and stored electronically, eliminating the need for a dark room, which not only saves space but also allows for easy transfer of images in a standard format. CR and DR technology may be a more expensive investment initially, but in the long run these technologies may be a cheaper alternative due to the elimination of film, film processors, chemicals, and facility space. Refurbished conventional equipment can be obtained fairly cheap, whereas new digital systems are available often costing significantly less than $100,000.

In addition to the imaging equipment technology, sites may require an archiving system that is often an additional expense. PACS allow for viewing, manipulation, and transfer of images. Imaging centers may require one or more PACS viewing stations. Obviously, PACS is required only if the site uses CR or DR technology.

As with the laboratory services, a complete cost analysis of imaging is required to assess potential revenue minus costs (i.e., labor, equipment, and supplies) in order to determine if the program is profitable and should be pursued. Preauthorization for testing may become a major issue for urgent care centers. This is less of an issue for EDs; however, retrospective denials can occur for these services. Medicare will likely expand scrutiny and may deny reimbursement of CT scans performed without appropriate justification and documentation. In addition, managed care contracts should be negotiated carefully with radiology services reimbursed as a carve-out from bundled services provided in the urgent care clinic if possible.

.: requirements

,gnificant space is required for all imaging equipment planned in the center. Leading of internal walls is required to reduce radiation exposure for patients and staff. Preplanning construction can reduce costs by using the outside walls of the center for the radiology or CT room, which reduces the amount of leading required with internal walls. For example, using the two outside corner walls of the clinic building for CT and radiology rooms reduces the leading needs from four to only two internal walls. Standard radiology rooms for musculoskeletal x-ray require approximately 300 square feet, and CT rooms require approximately 400 square feet of space.

CT scanning has resulted in dramatic changes in healthcare, with rapid diagnosis of many health problems. Space and power supply are important considerations when installing a CT scanner. Other testing modalities to consider in the development of an imaging center include ultrasound (which is also beneficial to the urgent care center), mammography, and bone density scanning. In addition to the listed equipment, as mentioned previously, PACS is an essential component that allows for ease of visualization, transfer, and storage of images. If digital mammography is being considered, images are often reviewed in real time by a radiologist to determine the need for additional imaging tests. This would require staffing an on-site radiologist and a complete radiology reading room.[7]

An imaging center is a costly endeavor and is often cost prohibitive to a single urgent care center. But many hospital-affiliated facilities have been successful by combining the urgent care and imaging centers. Figure 7.1 reviews average annual salaries of radiology department personnel, with the ultrasound tech having the highest salary, and Figure 7.2 provides a simple revenue estimate for procedures based on conservative Medicare rates.

FIGURE 7.1

CLINIC EMPLOYEES POSITION DESCRIPTION AND MEDIAN SALARY

POSITION	MEDIAN ANNUAL SALARY
Radiology technologist	$57,200
CAT scan technologist	$57,200
MRI technologist	$57,200
Ultrasound technologist	$70,500
Medical office manager	$83,500
Receptionist/clerical	$25,800

Source: State of Minnesota. (2011). Radiologic technologist: Illinois. Retrieved from http://www.careerinfonet.org/occ_rep.asp?next=occ_rep&Level=&optstatus=111111111&jobfam=29&id=1&nodeid=2&soccode=292034&stfips=17&x=54&y=8

FIGURE 7.2

PROJECTED IMAGING REVENUE

BASED ON VOLUME AND 7.5 HOURS OF TECHNICIAN TIME AND MEDICARE				
TEST	TIME/ MINUTES	MAXIMUM PER DAY	AVERAGE MEDICARE REVENUE	TOTAL REVENUE
Plain films	15	22.5	50	$1,125
Mammogram	30	15	100	$1,500
CT head	15	15	250	$3,750
CT other	30	7.5	350	$2,625
MRI	30	15	600	$9,000
Ultrasound	30	15	120	$1,800

Key Takeaway

Although laboratory and radiology services provide great benefits to any urgent care clinic, a complete cost analysis evaluating staffing, space, equipment, certification, recertification, oversight, and supplies for all options should be assessed using a simple Microsoft Excel–formatted spreadsheet to ensure that the cost of the service is less than the revenue generated to ensure financial viability of both the service and the clinic.

REFERENCES

1. Hale, T. 2012. Technology in Urgent Care: Digital or Conventional Imaging? J Urgent Care Med. 2012(4):18–19.

2. Dumas, T. An Urgent Care Lab as a Profit Center. J Urgent Care Med. 2011(2):18–25.

3. Weinick, R., Bristol, S., DesRoches, C. 2009. Urgent Care Centers in the U.S.: Findings from a National Survey. BMC Health Services Res. 9(1):79.

4. ibid.

5. Hale, T. 2012. Technology in Urgent Care: Digital or Conventional Imaging? J Urgent Care Med. 2012(4):18–19.

6. Beckman, H.B., et al. The Doctor-Patient Relationship and Malpractice: Lessons from Plaintiff's Depositions. Archives of Internal Medicine. 1994. 154(12): 1365.

7. Siegal, L. VA Design Guide Radiology Service. Retrieved 24 March 2012 from *www.wbdg.org/ccb/VA/VADEGUID/radio.pdf*. April 2008:1–111.

Clinical Patient Care Services

Our intent for this book is to assist administrators and medical professionals in evaluating the business potential of developing an urgent care center. There are ample textbooks that provide education on urgent care and emergency medicine. We do not cover clinical care protocols in detail, because this information can be easily found elsewhere, and we want to focus on some key aspects that require administrators to review. These aspects include expected medical complaints, potential extended medical treatment, minimum requirements for emergent care, treatment protocols, and medical staff requirements. Finally, we suggest some medical equipment that we have found make a significant impact for specific problems and help ease the care of the patient. The following are common clinical questions that administrators need to ask themselves:

- What is the most common diagnosis seen in an urgent care facility?

- What other conditions can be treated safely in an urgent care facility?

- Why would a clinic treat patients for prolonged periods of time?

- What emergencies should I prepare for?

Types of Clinical Care Treated

The majority of cases seen in urgent care clinics include minor medical complaints and injuries (see Figure 8.1). Most of these cases are managed without any diagnostics tests, and about 20%–25% require waive testing or radiographic studies while 2%–4% require both. Care for these minor complaints can be handled fairly quickly, which results in a much faster turnaround time than most emergency departments (ED). In our experience, treatment times range from an average of 60–90 minutes, which includes minor testing. These times are very competitive with private physician offices. Higher-risk diagnoses, including chest pain, abdominal pain, and headache, require a more extended evaluation period, which, in turn, prolongs turnaround times.

Extended care and high-risk complaints

As discussed in previous chapters, you will need to define the focus of your urgent care clinic and determine the extent of care that will be provided. Patients often

FIGURE 8.1

MINOR MEDICAL COMPLAINTS AND INJURIES

MEDICAL COMPLAINTS	INJURY
Cough/URI/bronchitis	Back pain/neck pain
Sore throat	Ankle/wrist sprains
Sinusitis	Extremity/facial/scalp lacerations
UTI	Contusions
Otitis media	
Conjunctivitis	

present with conditions such as asthma and can be easily cared for with multiple aerosols and steroids. If they improve after treatment, they can be discharged. This treatment frequently exceeds two hours, but it is billable at higher levels. Another diagnostic dilemma includes patients suffering from gastroenteritis with multiple episodes of vomiting and diarrhea. These patients, if otherwise healthy and younger, can often be cared for with appropriate antiemetic, such as ondansetron and one to two liters of intravenous (IV) fluids.

Both of these cases are examples of extended care that often requires two to three hours of clinic bed time. This extended treatment is billable and can increase reimbursement but does tie up clinic beds. If the urgent care clinic is hospital affiliated, providing extended workups and treatment can help reduce the burden on the ED. You can expand the clinical services, including abdominal pain, if you have the capability to do so. Many advanced-level urgent care clinics care for all acuity levels of patients but do not accept ambulance traffic.

Chest pain and abdominal pain are in the top five chief complaints for most EDs. These conditions require a complete evaluation with lab testing and radiographic studies. Expanding your urgent care clinic to this acuity level will significantly reduce bed turnover and should be considered only if you have adequate space, staffing, equipment, and technology. If you decide to treat higher-acuity patients, you need to ensure that you have the capability to do so, appropriate resuscitation equipment, and the ability to provide adequate, close follow-up care or transfer for hospital admission.

Chest pain is a very high-risk diagnosis that often requires serial EKGs, troponins, CT scanning (evaluating for pulmonary emboli), among other tests. Discharging a

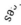

nt complaining of chest pain that may be cardiac in nature without provoca-
.: stress testing is a major risk. We strongly recommend transferring these
patients to the hospital or a very close follow-up for stress testing. Patients complaining of abdominal pain may be worked up in the clinic when ultrasound and
CT scanning are available. Even without a full-service lab, waived testing can
provide renal function results, allowing for performance of a contrasted CT scan.
Each center needs to determine the risk/benefit of providing extended evaluation
from a standpoint of flow, financial collections, and medical risk.

Medical Staff Issues

Most clinics do not maintain a list of medical staff or on-call physicians. But it is
a significant benefit to have relationships with specific subspecialty physicians,
including orthopedics and ophthalmology. Strong relationships with the local ED
and its medical director are also critical.

We have found that the need for orthopedic referral is essential, because the
majority of fractures require outpatient follow-up. Training staff on appropriate
splinting and stabilization techniques is not only necessary for good patient care
but also provides significant billable revenue. The following splints should provide
adequate stabilization of most fractures:

- Thumb spica

- Ulnar gutter splint

- Short arm splint/volar splint

- Long arm splint

- Sugar-tong splint posterior

- Posterior splint

- Stirrup splint

You should also maintain an adequate supply of moldable finger splints. Casting requires appropriate training to ensure there is enough room for swelling, which can be an issue if the cast is not applied appropriately. Casting also requires time. There are many commercial products using premolded splints with Velcro straps that make application fast and easy, but the costs of these splints are greater than the traditional "cut and mold" splints applied with an ace bandage. It is important that anyone applying splints understand that the classic moldable materials often become quite hot when activated with water, and they should take appropriate steps to avoid burning the skin. Protection and padding can be provided by cotton web roll. Splinting programs are available from many of the splinting supply venders who are more than happy to provide diagrams and educational DVDs. Local orthopedic physicians may also provide in-services on splinting if they are receiving referrals from your clinic.

Common eye complaints, especially with worker's compensation cases, include corneal foreign bodies. Most of these foreign bodies can be removed with the appropriate equipment, including a slit lamp. However, some may require corneal burring to remove rust rings that may not be available at the clinic, so you will need to refer them to an ophthalmologist.

Relationships with the local hospital ED make patient transfers much smoother. In addition, the urgent care center could serve as a referral site for the ED if structured correctly. If the center has a relationship with the hospitalist's program, patients who have an adequate workup can be directly admitted to the hospitalist service, bypassing the ED and avoiding prolonged waits.

Medical Emergencies

You should always hope for the best but plan for the worst. Each urgent care facility needs to determine what level of resuscitation equipment they should maintain on-site. This may depend on the proximity of EMS and ambulance transport. We recommend that medications include aspirin and epinephrine (for anaphylaxis). In addition, you should have a bag valve device with a mask to allow for ventilation in a cardiac arrest situation and have an automatic external defibrillator (AED) readily accessible. For a reasonable increased investment, the site could have a combined 12-lead EKG/monitor/defibrillator/pacer. These devices often include pulse oximetry and end tidal CO_2 monitoring. Many sites have a fully stocked "code cart" on-site with complete airway and resuscitation equipment. We have had each of the following occur on multiple occasions at our sites and suggest these steps be taken while waiting for the ambulance to arrive.

Anaphylaxis

1. If there are any problems with airway and breathing, you should support by opening the airway and assisting ventilation with a bag valve mask (insert airways if needed and available). Initiate CPR if needed and attach an AED if the patient is without pulse. The American Heart

Association now recommends chest compressions be started prior to airway insertion if the patient is unresponsive and without a pulse (see Basic Life Support Guidelines at *www.heart.org*).

2. Dial 911.

3. Obtain saline lock for IV access.

4. If a pulse is present and breathing is adequate, consider epinephrine subcutaneous or IV if anaphylaxis is present.

5. Transport by EMS to the ED.

Chest pain (if you are unable to provide an adequate evaluation at your site)

1. If there are any problems with airway and breathing, you should support by opening the airway and assisting ventilation with a bag valve mask (insert airways if needed and available). Initiate CPR if needed and attach an AED if the patient is without a pulse. The American Heart Association now recommends chest compressions be started prior to airway insertion if the patient is unresponsive and without a pulse (see Basic Life Support Guidelines at *www.heart.org*).

2. Dial 911.

3. If a pulse is present and breathing is adequate, consider giving aspirin if the patient is not allergic.

4.   Obtain a saline lock for IV access.

5.   Consider performing a 12-lead EKG and faxing or transmitting it to the ED for early identification of an acute myocardial infarction and cardiac cath lab activation.

6.   Transport by EMS to the ED.

Stroke symptoms

1.   If there are any problems with airway and breathing, you should support by opening the airway and assisting ventilation with a bag valve mask (insert airways if needed and available). Initiate CPR if needed and attach an AED if the patient is without a pulse. The American Heart Association now recommends chest compressions be started prior to airway insertion if the patient is unresponsive and without a pulse (see Basic Life Support Guidelines at *www.heart.org*).

2.   Dial 911.

3.   If a pulse is present and breathing is adequate, check blood sugar by finger stick and administer D50 if severely hypoglycemic.

4.   Obtain a saline lock for IV access.

5.   Consider performing a noncontrast head CT scan—only if this does not delay transport—especially if the urgent care center is part of the same

hospital system with PACS connectivity. This may decrease the time to thrombolytic therapy if indicated in the ED.

6. Transport by EMS to the ED with CT scan images or computer disc.

Active labor

1. If there are any problems with airway and breathing, you should support by opening the airway and assisting ventilation with a bag valve mask (insert airways if needed and available). Initiate CPR if needed and attach an AED if the patient is without a pulse. The American Heart Association now recommends chest compressions be started prior to airway insertion if the patient is unresponsive and without a pulse (see Basic Life Support Guidelines at *www.heart.org*).

2. Dial 911.

3. Obtain sterile gloves and evaluate the patient, with visual inspection of the patient's perineal area to determine if the patient is approaching delivery (crowning).

4. Obtain a saline lock for IV access.

5. Keep the mother comfortable.

6. Transport by EMS to the ED.

A Few Clinical Pearls of Wisdom

As I mature in my practice of medicine (I now have less hair and what's left is gray), I have developed a true respect for badness. Bad things can happen to good doctors and nice patients. The intent of this statement is not to scare clinicians but to remind them to always consider what the worst-case scenario could be. As discussed in the human resources chapter, emergency medicine trains physicians to think of what will kill my patient and work backward. Other specialists often consider what is the most likely diagnosis based on the presenting symptoms. Neither is incorrect, but they are different approaches and perspectives of practice.

The following are some clinical protocols to consider.

- Confusion, dizziness, and unexplained diaphoresis = finger stick blood sugar.

- Abdominal pain in females of childbearing age with a uterus (even if they have had a tubal ligation) = pregnancy test.

- Worst headache of life = transfer to ED or CT scan and, if the scan is normal, perform a spinal tap to ensure the patient does not suffer from a subarachnoid hemorrhage (or again transfer to ED).

- Chest pain = myocardial infarction until proven otherwise.

- Shortness of breath in adults (unless explainable, e.g., asthma) = EKG. You can decide on the age cutoff, but the bottom line is that acute myocardial infarctions are still the No. 1 killer of patients and represent the highest malpractice dollars in emergency medicine when this condition is missed or handled inappropriately. Don't assume the risk on these patients. Ship them to the ED.

The following are other lessons we have learned and personal opinions gained from experience.

- During influenza season, there will be one or more cases of pneumonia among all the standard flu cases. Consider getting a chest x-ray, especially if patients are older and have a low oxygen saturation (<95% is my number, but you can decide on your own).

- When there is a gastrointestinal (GI) bug going around, there is likely going to be one or more patients with appendicitis mixed in among all the cases of vomiting and diarrhea. If the patient presents with localized pain, consider the diagnosis. In addition, always tell patients they can come back if symptoms worsen. I also advise the majority of my patients with abdominal pain to be rechecked the next day, even if that means they need to come back to the ED or clinic. If it is the right thing for the patient, it's the right thing to do, period!

- You or colleagues will see, treat, and discharge:

  – A patient with reproducible chest pain and a "little" tachycardia who returns the next day with a pulmonary embolism (PE). Beware of the undiagnosed PE; this is a condition that is often missed and patients can, and do, die from pulmonary embolism. Consider using some screening criteria (Wells, etc., can be found at *www.medicalcriteria. com*) and include a D-dimer test based on the risk level. Somewhere in all those patients with cough, upper respiratory infection, bronchitis, asthma, and chronic obstructive pulmonary disorder, there is a patient with a missed PE. Please note that unexplained tachycardia in these types of patients may represent a PE. Always perform an initial complete set of vital signs, explain any abnormalities, and repeat vitals with a minimum of blood pressure and pulse on each patient at discharge—especially if the vitals were initally abnormal.

– A patient who got better with a GI cocktail only to return the next day with an acute MI (hopefully alive). Any patient you believe is at risk for an acute coronary syndrome should have an EKG performed and you should consider transferring to the ED for a workup if you cannot evaluate sufficiently. If they refuse to go, you must document it and explain to the patient that the risks of refusing treatment include death.

– The patient with the classic migraine, who has a long history of migraines and presents with a migraine that is just a little worse, is treated with your headache cocktail du jour. The patient improves only to return the next day with an intracerebral bleed. Document a complete neurologic exam on all headache patients and an assessment of nuchal signs (absence of rigidity). Consider scanning patients who present with a change in their pattern. In addition, a subarachnoid hemorrhage is not completely ruled out by a normal head CT. This is much less likely with the newer generation of CT scanners, but some patients still require an LP.

Key Takeaway

Even though urgent care centers treat many patients with minor complaints, you should always consider the worst-case scenario to protect your patients.

The center should be prepared for the occasional very ill patient. It is also an excellent practice to have strong relationships with both the local EMS agency/ rescue squad as well as the ED. Most cases will be handled with excellent care provided by your center. To prepare for emergency cases, make sure you have the right equipment and practice monthly for the unexpected. Being prepared means each team member understands their role in an emergency.

Patient Satisfaction: Creating and Delivering the Right Expectations

Most people have, on occasion, experienced remarkable customer service. Unfortunately, people tend to remember experiences of poor customer service much more clearly. People talk five times more frequently about poor experiences than favorable ones. But they will talk about a positive experience. Patients who encounter a problem during their urgent care visit who might complain later will most likely be satisfied if the problem is resolved on the spot. They'll also be surprised, which is why 95% of them will tell others (i.e., friends, family members, neighbors) about that positive experience. The difference between those patients—or customers—who are satisfied with their care in your urgent care center and those who are not is a critical indicator of how effectively your center carries out its mission. Consider the following customer service experience.

Seventeen years ago when I moved to eastern North Carolina, I was fortunate to find a female barber who I clearly felt had all of the professional characteristics of exemplary customer service. She had convenient hours of operation, so I could schedule appointments in the evening on a day when I was scheduled to be in town. Additional customer satisfaction characteristics included the following:

- Location: The salon was 5 minutes from my office and home.

- Hours: As noted, she maintained evening hours until 8 p.m. on three days during the week.

- Communication: The barber called to remind me of my scheduled appointment the Friday before, and if she had a cancellation during the day of the appointment she called me to determine if I wanted to come in earlier. She also routinely sent emails about her gardening, which was a hobby that we shared and discussed frequently.

So how could customer service get any better? And what would challenge my allegiance from this level of service?

The barber developed a chronic shoulder problem, which ultimately required surgery, and she was unable to work for nine months. She recommended two different barbers who agreed to help her with her clients during this surgery and recovery period. I tried them both, but was underwhelmed, due to the fact that they didn't keep evening hours or make reminder calls. I was discussing my disappointment in the new barbers with my wife (she may refer to this as whining) when she recommended I consider using the hair stylist she used.

The mere fact that my wife liked a hair stylist was sufficient credibility to the stylist's professional acumen and quality. In addition, my wife explained that Amy, the stylist, had a limited number of clients and made house visits rather than working from a salon. I was intrigued. So I scheduled an appointment for Amy to cut my hair in my office. It turned out that she was delayed and

20 minutes late, but she texted me to inform me of the delay beforehand and because I was at my office, the delay was irrelevant because it didn't interrupt my work. Amy is a self-contained professional and having my hair cut at my office was incredibly efficient. Her prices are consistent with other barbers; however, she earns a favorable margin because she has a much lower overhead burden, which allows her to limit her number of clients. I liked this solution.

Other aspects which made the experience favorable included the following:

- The option to receive text message communication rather than telephone calls. This was a plus to me because I am routinely on telephone calls, at client sites out of town, and not easily available due to travel and client meetings during the day. Amy responds to texting promptly and scheduling has been easy.

- Receiving barbering services at home or work is a tremendous improvement, because I am not burdened with travel or waiting time.

I am sold and love the new arrangement (and my wife never issued an "I told you so"; however, she reminded me to listen to her more often). It was hard for me to imagine that customer service could have gotten better than my first hair cutting arrangement. The following factors are what made this experience so outstanding:

- Courtesy: I was treated professionally, courteously, efficiently, and expeditiously. Amy already had an existing relationship with my wife and quickly determined what features would best meet my needs by discussing alternatives for communication, etc.

- Listening: My wife and Amy knew exactly what would work for me and, as many wives do, led me skillfully down the road, allowing me to think I was charting new territory.

- Informing: Texting works exceptionally well for me, and many times, I "piggy-back" an existing appointments at home when Amy is cutting my wife or boys' hair. Amy also texts my wife confirming my appointments.

- Concern: Amy routinely follows up with my wife and texts me for feedback on all appointments. Amy happens to be a gardener, as well, so again I have found someone to share a hobby with.

Now ask yourself: how well does your staff follow these types of practices with each patient in your urgent care site? They are, after all, your customers. Doing everything you can to ensure that they are happy with the service you are providing is critical to running a successful urgent care center. When your patients are not happy, your business will suffer because they will choose to receive care elsewhere.

The Cost of Dissatisfied Patients

No one likes to hear complaints about the service they provide. But you should remember that the vast majority of dissatisfied customers never complain, which means that complaint is only the tip of the iceberg. For every patient who is unhappy with the service in your urgent care center and complains, there are six other patients who were equally disappointed. Even though they may not complain to you, you can be sure they are complaining to other people. On average, they will relate the experience to 8 to 10 other people. Now you have roughly 63 people who have heard about the negative encounter. As a result, about one in four will decide not to seek treatment at your urgent care center. An average revenue of $200 per visit and an average of five lifetime visits per patient, the total revenue lost from these 16 patients is $16,000. And that's just for one complaint.

But you're not done losing money yet. When a patient complains, you have to handle that complaint, which entails costs. The average urgent care complaint requires $375 in costs to the center. For a center with an average number of complaints—around 52 per year—the cost of dealing with these complaints amounts to $19,500 annually.

Historic context

Twenty-five years ago when prospective healthcare administrators were learning strategies to evaluate healthcare services, their training focused on five primary characteristics:

1. Access to care

2. Continuity of care

3. Comprehensiveness of care

4. Quality of care

5. Cost-effectiveness of care

Customer service didn't even make the list. Patient satisfaction, if considered at all, was placed under quality of care. Times have definitely changed. If you analyze that list in the context of urgent care, customer satisfaction rises even higher on it now than it has risen in many other areas.

The obvious component in access to care—being able to reach a facility that provides emergency care—is available for most people. Another part of access, and a characteristic that was considered 25 years ago, is choice—the ability to choose between different facilities. Few individuals wake up in the morning and set this goal: My day will be fulfilled if I achieve a visit to the urgent care clinic. People end up at urgent care sites because of circumstances beyond their control. Access to care, in the sense of choice, is in effect moot in regard to emergency care. Continuity of care, although obviously very important, is usually more of a factor beyond the urgent care clinic when patients transfer. Comprehensiveness of care is a critical factor and involves coordination of healthcare professional team members' efforts within the center. However, coordination goes on mostly behind the scenes. And to the extent that patients notice, it is closely related to their perception of customer service—positive or negative. Clearly, quality is essential, and it is tied closely with their perception of customer service. Cost-effectiveness is assumed by most patients who visit an urgent care center.

In the past 25 years, more emphasis has been placed on healthcare professionals' responsibility and role in improving the patient's satisfaction. Increasingly, this emphasis has been driven by economic reasons, by regulatory agencies imposing minimally accepted standards of service, and by consumers themselves who demand better service and who have more information about healthcare conditions immediately accessible, especially from the Internet, than in years past. Urgent care is a visible arena, where customer satisfaction or dissatisfaction significantly affects community perception about the center. As a result, urgent care owners must focus on customer satisfaction to remain competitive.

Competition and consumer demand are among the primary differences in how we evaluated healthcare services 25 years ago versus today. (See Figure 9.1.)

FIGURE 9.1

CHANGES IN EVALUATING PROVISION OF HEALTHCARE SINCE 1985

25 YEARS AGO	NOW
Medical staff (private attending physicians) generates ≥75% of hospital admissions, and many private physician offices—were open or available seven days per week	Emergency departments often generate ≥75% of hospital inpatient admissions (private attending physicians opt to have hospitalists provide inpatient care). Urgent care centers have supplied the access that private practices no longer provide—most are open seven days per week with extended evening hours.
Very little competition	Tremendous competition (both from other providers and ever increasingly from financial pressures to remain viable).
Managed care payers or payer contracts do not define care standards	Payer agreements define specific care standards and impose penalties for not meeting care standards (customer satisfaction components included).
Physician identified as the primary customer	Physician shares the identity of primary customer with patient and payer.

Improving Patient Satisfaction

The following are four steps that can improve patient satisfaction:

- Reduce wait times

- Make structural changes

- Manage perceptions and expectations

- Analyze patient satisfaction surveys and complaints

We often equate customer service to just being nice rather than involving a deep exploration of what the customer values in the urgent care encounter. For example, structural change refers to improving the cleanliness and the appearance of the waiting room, ensuring privacy in the registration area, making blankets and pillows available, and providing comfortable chairs. You need to really analyze surveys and complaints to identify factors that lead to patient satisfaction or the lack thereof. Most centers simply respond to particular survey points rather than embed customer satisfaction as an integral part of their urgent care processes.

Ask the patients—and tell the clinicians

Urgent care centers are similar to a restaurant in that their clients make a choice to visit the center. We strongly recommend that urgent care sites routinely survey their patients to gauge the extent to which desired attributes of patient satisfaction were present, as well as patients' overall perception of their experience.

What do these surveys ask patients and does your staff know? Is your staff aware of the survey results? We have consulted with urgent care sites throughout the United States, and we are continually surprised by how few physicians, nurses, and other midlevel providers have seen an actual copy of the patient satisfaction survey upon which their performance is judged. The survey should be an open-book test, and all professionals involved in providing care at urgent care sites should know what questions the patient will be asked. Besides providing your team a copy of the survey, owners should also hold discussion and coaching sessions and coordinate these efforts so the entire team can focus its efforts on improving a patient's experience. Remember our example of hair cutting and how communication, including expectations, and minimal handoffs were well coordinated.

Patient satisfaction surveys usually focus on the following four main topics:

- Courtesy

- How much time the staff took to listen to the patient

- How well informed the patient was about the treatment

- The doctor, nurse practitioner, or physician assistant's concern about the patient's comfort

Urgent care may have an unusual context for expectations of customer service, but they are essentially the same as our reflections on why the hair cutting experience was positive. Keep that example in mind as we look at these four themes in urgent care. (We'll use doctors in our discussion, but it applies to nurses and other staff members on the healthcare team as well.)

Courtesy of the staff

Courtesy is a fundamental component of effective human communication. Verbal aspects of interaction between healthcare providers and patients demonstrate the truth of this assertion. However, nonverbal behavior is also significant. If the patient observes the physician looking at the clock or a wristwatch, the patient forms an impression of his or her relative importance to the physician, and they probably won't rate the doctor's courtesy highly. The urgent care manager should help doctors see how they're perceived by sharing comments from patients on surveys that offer insight on the interactions. The more closely the comments can be tied to real interactions with actual patients so that doctors can re-create the interaction, the more beneficial this sharing will be.

Taking time to listen

Patients' perception of this characteristic depends not only on the actual time spent in the interaction but in the quality of the communication. Once again, nonverbal behavior plays a crucial role in forming the patient's perception about how much time the doctor took to listen. If the doctor sits down when speaking with the patient, then the perception is usually that the doctor has taken more time even if the actual duration isn't any different than if the doctor had remained standing. How involved the patient is allowed to be in the conversation is another important factor in the patient's perception of how well the doctor listened. Remember that perception forms not just from the actual duration of time spent but also from the content of the communication.

Informing the patient

How well informed the patient feels depends not only on what information the doctor provides but also on how the doctor provides it. Did the physician include expectations of how the treatment will proceed and what it will accomplish? How other members of the healthcare team reinforced this information also helps determine the patient's perception. Informing the patient is a challenge to many healthcare professionals, because of the barriers erected by the use of medical terminology—acronyms, abbreviations, and "medicalese" in general. Hospitals, in this regard, are often not user-friendly to the public, and this is an opportunity for the urgent care center to differentiate itself by ensuring that the entire staff is oriented to language the patient and family will understand.

Concern for comfort

People don't go to an urgent care clinic unless they have to, and pain is usually the reason patients are there. A key part of the patient's perception about the quality of treatment is how well the doctor or nurse understands their level of pain and how adequately the team member responds to ameliorate it. Patients need to feel heard, need to understand the process for assessing their condition, and need to understand what latitude the doctor has to reduce their pain.

Specific Techniques to Satisfy Your Patients

We recommend using scripts to address the overall satisfaction of patients with their experience in your urgent care center. This approach can increase the likelihood that patients will recommend your center to others. These scripts contain specific wording intended to address the patients' concerns we've been discussing. Often, more experienced doctors, nurses, and other team members can provide the content to less experienced professionals. Contributing to an overall impression of care are the following behaviors:

- Complete explanations

- Promptness

- Friendliness and caring

- Putting patients at ease

- Providing updates and feedback

The patient's experience begins when that person arrives at the center, and the factors involved in creating satisfaction start immediately: for instance, the wait time before the patient's arrival is noticed, helpfulness of the first person encountered, comfort of the waiting area, the wait time to reach the treatment area, and then the wait time to see the doctor. To improve patient satisfaction during these initial stages, you can ensure that the reception and waiting areas are clean; provide frequent updates; set expectations for the patient early; offer diversions in the waiting room for all age groups, including a play area for young children, health-network television, and educational materials; post or otherwise communicate waiting times; and provide refreshments for companions of patients. You should drill into your staff's consciousness this goal: Door-to-doctor time should be 10 minutes 80% of the time.

Another aspect that impacts the patient's satisfaction is capturing and verifying personal insurance information. It is important to treat patients with courtesy and provide them privacy during the collection of this information. The ease of giving this information is also important.

After that introductory phase, initial contact between team members and the patient forms the all-important first impression of the treatment process. Your doctors, nurses, and other professionals should practice the following behaviors that reinforce the positive tone you should already have established in the first phase, such as:

- Knock before entering

- Recognize the patient's concern about time

- Thank the patient for waiting

- Introduce yourself to everyone in the room

- Acknowledge the patient's concerns

- Demonstrate caring and respect for privacy

- Explain transitions

The closing phase of the patient's encounter is just as important as the initial greeting. Make sure the discharge process is simple and understandable. Coach staff members to use scripts to clarify expectations of service in this process and resolve problems.

Getting to know the staff

You shouldn't underestimate the importance of setting the right tone from the beginning. But the central phase that establishes the conditions for satisfying patients is the behavior of your healthcare professionals in treating them. For physicians, the key aspects are the doctor's courtesy, whether the doctor took time to listen and inform the patient of what to expect with treatment, and the doctor's concern for the patient's comfort. Coach your doctors to keep the patients informed, introduce themselves properly, sit with the patients whenever possible, conduct an exit visit whenever possible, use scripts, and attend to the patient's pain and general comfort.

For nurses, the expectations are similar and include their courtesy to patients and their families and friends, whether they took time to listen and inform patients and their families and friends, their attention to patients' needs, their concern for privacy, and whether they let family and friends stay with patients. Train and mentor your nurses on how to use scripts, be aware of comfort and caring concerns, frequently contact patients and families and explain treatment and transitions, check in every hour to see whether they need blankets and pillows, and make contact every 15 minutes.

In regard to your technicians as well as nurses, significant factors are the courtesy of the person who draws blood and concern over the patient's comfort during this procedure, wait time for radiology tests, courtesy of the radiology staff, and concern for comfort during those tests.

Helping to resolve problems as they're occurring is also important for management. Staff members should be trained to resolve problems while they're occurring by rehearsing potential situations. Providing buttons to staff members that read "Ask me" or "May I help you?" and business cards are simple tools that help reinforce your staff members' efforts to satisfy their patients. Administrators should ensure that there is follow-up contact by phone for every patient who leaves the urgent care center to be transferred to an ED and for every pediatric patient within 24 hours.

Administrators should track patient satisfaction scores, compliments, and complaints by provider. Celebrate accomplishments in customer service. Train staff members in survival skills and reinforce them. Conduct patient focus groups, and selectively use secret shoppers to test the quality of customer service in your urgent care center.

Management should be sensitive to satisfaction not just of patients but of another group: staff members.

Quality Issues

Consider specific methods to enhance customer satisfaction during various phases of treatment but make sure that you reinforce key behaviors that staff members should always practice with patients regardless of the patients' stage of treatment. These include providing complete explanations; being prompt, friendly, and caring; putting patients at ease; and providing updates and feedback.

Remember that patients always want to be informed about delays throughout their entire urgent care encounter. They want to feel like the staff members care about them as people, and they want to have their pain controlled. They want to receive information about home care that they understand, and they want to feel safe in the center.

PATIENT WAITING

One experience we all share all too often in modern life is waiting in line. The psychology of waiting concerns how we perceive different aspects of that experience. From studies delving into the psychology of waiting, organizations have developed methods to manage waits and exploit findings on our perceptions. Businesses, in particular, have made good use of those methods. When you are unable to avoid a queue, understanding the principles derived from the studies and applying the methods help enhance patients' perceptions of flow and thus increase patient satisfaction. In a sense, you're inducing artificial flow—but doing so is okay in this context. There is a lot of excellent material available on the psychology of waiting, some of which we've discussed in Jensen et al. 2007 and Mayer and Jensen 2009.[1,2] The following are some of the principles first identified by David Maister in 1985.[3]

Time with nothing to do seems longer

When you're behind two grocery carts loaded with items at the checkout counter, time seems to drag forever. You have nothing to do other than stare at the candy or tabloids. If, on the other hand, you've ever been in line at the Star Tours ride at Walt Disney World, you probably recall winding your way through a building with androids in various states of repair, exotic machines, and realistic props, creating the impression that you're inside an enormous hangar in the *Star Wars* galaxy and leaving you so absorbed that you may actually regret moving too fast past some props. You may actually wait 15 minutes in the grocery line and 30 minutes in the Disney queue, but the former seems twice as long as the latter. To take a simpler example, restaurants often provide waiting customers with menus to look over before their table is ready or direct them to the bar, where there is usually a television with sporting events on. We tend to perceive waiting when we have nothing to occupy the time as dragging on longer than when we can concentrate on something interesting.

We can put the same principle to work in urgent care centers. Providing magazines to read and a television to watch gives patients something to do while they wait. Filling

PATIENT WAITING (CONT.)

out necessary forms as part of registration does too. The more patients perceive that they have something interesting to pass the time while they're waiting, the more satisfied they'll be. Allowing them to have family members or friends wait with them helps them pass the time more pleasantly.

A similar perception makes us think that if we get started in an activity quickly, the entire activity goes more quickly than when we have to wait longer to begin, even if the overall time spent in the activity is similar. We can take advantage of this perception in the center by using tools that improve flow anyway, such as triage, team triage, and sending patients directly to a room. You keep patient satisfaction high while you smooth flow. Moving patients sequentially also gives them a sense that they are in process, so if patients go from triage to registration to a room, the time seems to pass more quickly than if they're just waiting in the entrance area to be seen by anyone.

Uncertainty makes waiting seem longer

If your flight has been delayed and you start to worry about making a connection, you can get pretty anxious. Having to wait increases that anxiety. Uncertainty about how long you're going to have to wait makes time seem to drag as well. And unexplained delays also create the perception of time dragging. If a representative of the airline tells you what caused the delay of your flight and when you're likely to be able to leave, your anxiety level goes down. Patients encountering delays often get anxious too, and the principle for responding to that anxiety is the same: Let your patients know why delays have occurred. Regular contact with patients waiting eases their anxiety and makes the time seem to pass more quickly. Letting your patients know when they're likely to be treated and what the process will consist of provides more certainty, which in turn helps patients' perception of time passing. If a major trauma case is occupying multiple resources, explaining why patients are waiting longer helps manage perception. Most people are likely to understand when you explain delays to them in this kind of situation.

PATIENT WAITING (CONT.)

Fairness and value

If someone cuts in that grocery line in front of you, that action triggers your sense of injustice. And when you feel your wait is unfair, it seems longer. Be aware of this perception in designing your processes and the layout of your urgent care center. The farther apart you can keep different groups of people likely to proceed at different speeds through the center, the better you'll be able to maintain patient satisfaction. If someone waiting sees someone else who entered the center after him or her headed to the fast track, a sense of inequitable treatment is likely to arise. Communication is important here, too; the more you communicate with patients waiting, explaining why someone else went ahead, the better you can manage these perceptions.

Other perceptions arise from a sense of value. If you get on the waiting list for dinner at an exclusive restaurant known for its great cuisine, waiting an hour for a table may seem a small inconvenience and well worth enduring. Waiting an hour at your ordinary neighborhood burger joint, on the other hand, is likely time you're not willing to spend. The healthcare system is no different from restaurants in this regard. If your center has a reputation as the best in the area, with excellent care and customer service, patients will very likely submit to waiting longer without complaint. People are willing to wait longer if they perceive quality to be high. You want to enhance flow, of course, so waiting is minimized, but achieving excellence in many aspects reinforces the quality and effectiveness of all aspects of your operation.

Keeping company

If you've ever waited by yourself for an appointment, say for a job interview, you know that time spent waiting can really seem to drag. If you're waiting in a public area and end up talking with the people around you, the time seems to pass more quickly. In the urgent care center, you can manage this perception by making sure patients can wait with family members or friends. Regular contact helps mitigate the perception of time dragging as well. If you are communicating regularly with patients who are waiting,

---

PATIENT WAITING (CONT.)

those waiting by themselves will feel less isolated. If you can figure out how to make the general atmosphere in the waiting areas of your urgent care center enhance communication between strangers, you'll help reduce the sense of waiting alone and thus help make the passage of time seem shorter.

Source: Adapted from *The Healthcare Executive's Guide to Emergency Department Management*. HealthLeaders Media.[4]

Key Takeaway

It takes a team to improve patient satisfaction. Urgent care physicians or nurse practitioners are often the most visible members of the staff to patients. These clinicians also lead the efforts of all the staff members involved in treating your patients. They set the tone and can make a huge impact in assisting the rest of the staff, but they can't do it all themselves. Remember the group treating your patients is a team, and achieving high levels of patient satisfaction requires that your staff functions effectively as a team. If the doctor is not effectively setting the right tone, the rest of the team will have great difficulty overcoming that poor attitude. On the other hand, if the entire team works in a well-coordinated fashion in which roles and responsibilities are well defined and the team has a shared commitment to helping each patient efficiently and effectively and in a caring, courteous fashion, patients get better and the people caring for the patients receive additional rewards for a job well done.

Chapter 9

REFERENCES

1. Jensen, K., Mayer, T., Welch, S., Haraden, C. 2007. Leadership for Smooth Patient Flow. Health Administration Press, Chicago, IL.

2. Mayer, T., Jensen, K. 2009. Hardwiring Flow: Systems and Processes for Seamless Patient Care. Firestarter Publishing, Gulf Breeze.

3. Maister, D. 1984. The Psychology of Waiting Lines. Harvard Business Online, April.

4. Jensen, K., Kirkpatrick, D. 2011. The Healthcare Executive's Guide to Emergency Department Management. HealthLeaders Media.

Marketing Strategies

Marketing your urgent care center is an essential component to establishing name recognition, achieving your business objectives, and, in some cases, supporting the parent organization. We will examine both the commonalities and differences in marketing the various models of urgent care centers: retail centers, cash clinics, full-service urgent care centers, and freestanding emergency departments (ED).

The fundamental starting point in establishing a marketing plan requires a comprehensive exploration of the business purpose behind your urgent care model, so you can compile your marketing objectives. The following list will help you define the business aspects of your urgent care center, so you can develop a sound marketing plan.

1. **Outline the product or service.** You need to fully understand what it is you're offering, to whom, when, and why.

2. **Understand your market.** You need to know who your customers are to ensure that they not only know about but also will access your services. You should develop strategies on how you will break into this market in year one, as well as years three and five.

3.   **Define your goals.** You should establish 6-, 12-, and 18-month goals into service delivery to help you define success. It is important to know your target market segment and what volumes you expect to achieve, both quantitative in numbers and dollars and collections.

4.   **Know your service delivery team.** It is important to know which staff has the best potential to represent your service, impact the market you intend to tap into, and successfully achieve patient satisfaction.

5.   **Develop a marketing budget and business plan.** Force yourself through the discipline and rigor of developing your marketing plans and monitoring actual performance against your plans. This will allow you to quickly assess when performance deviates from what you anticipated. This doesn't necessarily indicate a right or wrong step, rather an opportunity for both short- and long-term adjustments. (See Figure 10.1 for an urgent care center business plan.)

Tailoring the Marketing Message

As we identified earlier in the book, urgent care centers, retail clinics, cash clinics, and freestanding EDs focus on service delivery to less acute patients in need of immediate, or perceived immediate, medical attention. It has been well established that female household members generally between 25 and 55 years of age are the primary healthcare decision-makers in the United States. Therefore, the marketing message should be easily understood and fashioned for this healthcare decision-maker.

FIGURE 10.1

SAMPLE URGENT CARE BUSINESS PLAN

Urgent Care - SAMPLE

				Visit	
Revenue				15,000.00	
Annual Visits				15,000.00	
Urgent Care - SAMPLE	$ 1,728,750.00		$	115.25	
	$ 1,728,750.00				
Deductions	$ 414,900.00		Deductions	24.00%	
Net Revenue		$ 1,313,850.00			
Expenses					
Billing		$ 105,108.00	Billing @ 8% Revenue		
Non-Provider Salaries	$ 311,064.00				
Provider Salaries	$ 364,000.00				
Leave Replacement	$ 67,506.40				
Salaries		$ 742,570.40			
Benefits		$ 163,365.49	Benefits @ 22%		
Materials & Supplies		$ 65,692.50	5% Net Revenue		
Rent		$ 60,000.00	4000 @ $15 ft sq		
Utilities		$ 8,000.00			
Cleaning/Maintenance		$ 8,000.00	$2 sq ft including maint agrmnts		
Telephone		$ 8,000.00			
Recruitment		$ 10,000.00	20000 for MD 10000 for PA		
Advertising		$ 39,415.50	3% of Revenue		
Accounting		$ 12,000.00			
Automobile		$ 2,000.00	6000 miles		
Bank Charges		$ 4,800.00	$400 mos		
Business Meals		$ 6,000.00	$500 mos		
Continuing Education		$ 5,000.00			
Management Fee		$ 65,692.50	5% of Net Revenues		
Consultants		$ 10,000.00			
Dues & Subscription		$ 2,000.00			
Insurance					
Malpractice	$ 15,000.00				
General Liability	$ 5,000.00	$ 20,000.00			
Lab Fees		$ 13,138.50	1% Revenue		
Licenses		$ 500.00			
Legal		$ 5,000.00			
Payroll Service		$ 1,600.00			
NC Franchise Tax		$ 1,200.00			
Personal Property Tax		$ 2,500.00			
Travel		$ 5,000.00			
Transcription		$ 5,000.00			
Total Expenses		$ 1,371,582.89			

FIGURE 10.1

SAMPLE URGENT CARE BUSINESS PLAN (CONT.)

Urgent Care - SAMPLE **Staffing**

	Hrs/Wk	FTEs	Staff	Annual Hrs	Wage	
Registration/Front Desks	116	2.9	2 Staff	6032	$ 8.50	$ 51,272.00
RNs		0	1.5 Staff	0	$ 20.00	$ -
LPNs	76	1.9	2 Staff	3952	$ 15.00	$ 59,280.00
X-ray Tech	76	1.9	1 Staff	3952	$ 16.00	$ 63,232.00
Office Mgr	40	1	1 Staff	2080	$ 27.00	$ 56,160.00
Case Manager	20	0.5	1 Staff	1040	$ 20.00	$ 20,800.00
Administrative Assistant	20	0.5	1 Staff	1040	$ 10.00	$ 10,400.00
Lab Tech	40	1	1 Staff	2080	$ 14.00	$ 29,120.00
Marketing	20	0.5	1 Staff	1040	$ 20.00	$ 20,800.00
		10.2				$ 311,064.00
MD	80	2	1 Staff	4160	$ 70.00	$ 291,200.00
PA	40	1	1 Staff	2080	$ 35.00	$ 72,800.00
						$ 364,000.00

FIGURE 10.1

SAMPLE URGENT CARE BUSINESS PLAN (CONT.)

Urgent Care - SAMPLE   **CAPITAL PLAN**

		Per	Total
Need 10 exam rooms		$ 10,000.00	$ 100,000.00
2 rooms more expensive			
Lab Equipment		$ 10,000.00	$ 10,000.00
PCs		$ 2,000.00	$ 20,000.00
EKG		$ 5,000.00	$ 5,000.00
Hearing Test		$ 3,000.00	$ 3,000.00
X-ray		$ 25,000.00	$ 25,000.00
Furniture			
desks	5	$ 1,000.00	$ 5,000.00
chairs	40	$ 100.00	$ 4,000.00
desk chairs	10	$ 200.00	$ 2,000.00
lamps	4	$ 250.00	$ 1,000.00
TVs	2	$ 750.00	$ 1,500.00
decorations			$ 10,000.00
breakroom			$ 2,500.00
Equipment			
copy			$ 10,000.00
fax			$ 500.00
telephone system			$ 25,000.00
file cabinets	10	$ 300.00	$ 3,000.00
chart rack			$ 10,000.00
signage			$ -
scales	2	$ 250.00	$ 500.00
Supply stock			$ 25,000.00
Miscellaneous			$ 50,000.00
			$ 313,000.00
Funding A/R (2 months at $200,000)			$ 400,000.00

The following questions can help ensure that your marketing is aimed toward the primary decision-maker.

1. How does your service delivery build on the decision-maker's existing trust and confidence?

2. Are your services convenient for this healthcare decision-maker?

3. How do you provide not just an acceptable but the preferred continuum of care for the healthcare decision-maker?

4. How do your services meet the decision-maker's expectations in terms of delivering high-quality and cost-effective care?

5. How do you provide comprehensive (one-stop shopping) to ensure that the healthcare decision-maker receives acceptable, or preferred, evaluation, treatment, and follow-up care?

It is vital to understand how your urgent care center fits within your broader continuum of care when you are defining both expectations and the marketing message. For the acute care hospital seeking to add urgent care services to an existing continuum of care, it is essential that they work with the medical staff to develop and offer the service as a supplement to existing medical and clinic practices. For the physician developing an urgent care center, it is imperative that the center be located in an area to achieve accessibility, have the support of other medical practices that will help establish confidence and trust in the eyes of the healthcare decision-makers, and be launched on the reputation of credible practitioners. For those seeking to develop the retail clinic and cash clinics, building the service delivery on the "coattails" of existing retail operations (i.e., pharmacies and clinics) increases the potential of a successful retail clinic operation.

Building the Marketing Plan

The marketing plan for hospital-affiliated urgent care centers should be complementary to the hospital or health system to expand its market share and market convenience. To do so, the urgent care center marketing plan should be developed with the same rigor questioning market analysis and plan development the healthcare system undergoes for its short- and longer-term planning and public relations and community relations.

For the retail centers and cash clinics, the owners must impose the same rigor in developing their marketing plan as they do in developing their business plan. Consequently, these sites should develop a plan defining pre-startup promotional activities, such as opening activities and announcements, and follow-up activities to nurture relationships with primary care physicians and community hospitals.

The fundamentals of heightened patient satisfaction and customer service as identified in Chapter 9 should be the primary objectives for patient service delivery from which a positive and favorable reputation will be forged.

Key concepts for promotional consideration should include:

- Involvement in community healthcare screenings (vision, diabetes, prostate screening, high school athletic exams, and occupational fitness, etc.).

- Advertising for evening and weekend hours as a supplement to physician practices. Pediatricians should be enlisted to refer patients or families to the urgent care center for afterhours care, primary care practitioners should be enlisted to refer patients to the urgent care center on weekends for immediate attention, etc.

- Community organizations that are actively involved with healthcare decision-makers should be targeted both for advertisement and presentations, e.g., PTAs, civic organizations, and churches.

- Opportunities to have a question-and-answer column in the local newspaper can effectively heighten awareness of the urgent care center.

- Soliciting patient testimonials describing patient care that exceeded the consumer's expectations should be solicited and promoted both through brochures and letters in the waiting room and incorporated into flyers or advertisements.

- All urgent care center staff should undergo rigorous and continued customer satisfaction training and coaching to ensure that each customer encounter exceeds core expectations.

- Consideration should be given for allowing use of the urgent care center facility when not in service, i.e., during certain hours the lobby may be used for civic purposes or support groups or other social meeting needs.

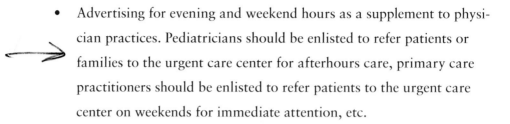

Marketing Basics

Essential methods of marketing include word of mouth, physician referrals, appropriate signage (including billboards), ZIP code–targeted mailers, and the Internet and websites.

Word-of-mouth marketing is usually accomplished by having great customer service. Engaging local primary care and specialist physicians, so they verbally refer patients to your facility, can be accomplished by meeting with each provider one on one and describing that your site is for episodic care and can serve as an afterhours alternative for the physician's office. You can suggest that service will be outstanding and more cost-effective than the local ED. You should also commit to provide visit information back to the physician practice (with appropriate patient permission). You could even suggest that the practice's afterhours voice message can recommend your site for appropriate minor care rather than suggesting the ED. In addition, you can suggest that the clinic will refer patients who are in need of primary care to these same practices.

Signage is a key element in the success of your center. It should specifically state that you provide urgent medical care, if allowed by your state. If the center is located near a freeway, billboard advertising will help market your services to thousands of drivers. The billboard should be close to the site and should include the phrase: "Urgent Medical Care This Exit" (again, if allowed by state regulations).

As most consumers now use the Internet, you should have your information about your center in cyberspace by developing a website. There are many vendors who can provide assistance with improving traffic to your website that should translate into increased visits to your center at a very reasonable price.

And remember, patients aren't your only customers. Managed care organizations (MCO) are customers as well and they play a major role in where patient seek treatment (see Chapter 5). You can improve business from MCOs by marketing directly to these companies and becoming a preferred provider for urgent care services. MCOs are looking for urgent care clinics to do the following:

1. Have afterhours, weekend, and holiday care

2. Obtain urgent care center certification (see *www.UCAOA.org*)

3. Strongly consider accreditation through the Joint Commission (*www.jointcommission.org*)

4. Provide basic radiology services (plain x-rays at minimum)

Key Takeaway

Marketing is a critical cost of doing business. The best marketing is through word of mouth and outstanding patient experience. Providing afterhours services for local medical practices helps to build your business. Becoming involved in community events and marketing to public organizations also can help the clinic's image and increase patient volume. Signage at the site and billboard use should ct vehicular traffic to your site. Finally, professional websites with continued ring, updating, and improvement can capture Internet-savvy patients.

Safety and Risk Management

Healthcare professionals want to provide high-quality, reliable, compassionate service. Healthcare organizations that consistently achieve high-quality outcomes are not concerned only with how well they are doing. They are also concerned with what can potentially go wrong at any time. In fact, they are obsessed with it. These organizations focus continually on what can go wrong and how to fix or, better yet, prevent it. The key is to prevent errors as much as possible. Still, errors occur every day in our urgent care centers. You need to accept this fact and move toward reducing the frequency of errors and preventing harm when errors do occur. And this last goal, after all, is what we're really seeking: Preventing patient harm, not just preventing errors.

A Culture of Safety

The following are five principles of reliability and safety that you should consider before we talk about handling errors and how to prevent harm.

1. All people make mistakes

2. "First, do no harm" does not mean "do not make any mistakes"

3.   Most error-prone or high-risk situations are predictable, manageable, and preventable

4.   A strong culture of safety is essential

5.   A collaborative approach results in better outcomes, and an organization's preoccupation with failure is essential

A culture of safety focuses on reducing errors, predicting what may go wrong, learning from errors that do happen, and preventing harm when errors occur. A culture of safety makes errors visible when they do occur and then mitigates their impact.

You can predict patient volume, patient acuity, and patient demand for specific services. And you can smooth flow to produce a more effective process, one that will reduce the likelihood of errors. The lessons on teamwork apply equally well in this context, because teamwork and communication enable you to establish an effective collaborative atmosphere. In a collaborative culture of safety, you don't play the blame game. In the old peer review and quality-assurance models, you stressed who was at fault. In new collaborative models, you convey clearly to team members that you understand they do not come to work to make errors and you want to minimize the risk as much as they do.

A systematic approach

You can't attain a 100% error-free operation. Many people throughout your organization make errors, not just a few who stand out. This lesson implies something important: You should emphasize systems rather than individuals.

In an article on errors in medicine in 1994, Lucien Leape noted that the 197 accident at the Three Mile Island nuclear power plant in Pennsylvania caused psychologists and human-factors engineers to reexamine their theories about human error. Many of the errors that led to the Three Mile Island incident were caused by faulty interface design, others by complex interactions and breakdowns that neither operators nor their instruments could detect.[1] Disasters of this magnitude, such as the Bhopal chemical explosion in India and the nuclear accident at Chernobyl in the Soviet Union, resulted from a series of major failures due to organizational design that occurred long before the accident—failures that caused operator errors and made them impossible to reverse.

Faulty processes account for 85% of problems in a system, and human inadequacy only 15% of problems. Urgent care centers are not much different from other healthcare facilities in this regard. Charles Vincent and his colleagues pioneered the use of an investigative process for medical accidents in which hospital staff members comprehensively examine all factors that could be involved. Invariably, they report that this process uncovers multiple system defects and reveals clearly that accidents result from multiple causes of which the obvious human error is often the least important.[2] Robust systems of any kind anticipate common cognitive errors and build in safeguards to identify and counteract them before they affect vital processes.

When errors do happen, if you use a systems approach, you view them as resources. Adverse events, near misses, and errors waiting to happen are opportunities to learn about the system—and near misses reveal weaknesses in the system just as effectively as errors but at a much lower cost in human misery and wasted resources. Errors and near misses provide the data for a systemic approach to preventing adverse events. After an error occurs, ask two questions:

1. Why did this mistake happen?

2. What redesign would make this error less likely?

A culture of safety focuses on measures of process, gained as you work to improve flow. Studying human performance has the potential to help organizations continually improve system of care and reduce bad outcomes due to errors.

T. W. Nolan describes three ways to increase the safety and reliability of a medical system[3]:

1. Design the system to prevent errors

2. Design procedures to make errors visible when they do occur so they can be intercepted

3. Design procedures for mitigating the adverse effects of errors when they are not detected and intercepted

 Nolan suggests several actions to achieve these three goals: Reduce complexity, optimize information processing, automate wisely, use constraints, and mitigate unwanted side effects of change. The more you can simplify and the more steps you can eliminate from your processes, the more likely you will be able to reduce potential errors in the system.

PREVENTING HARM

To establish a culture of safety in your urgent care center, keep the following nine principles in mind:

- Hire the right team

- Emphasize teamwork and communication

- Implement after-action reviews

- Emphasize error reporting

- Manage high-risk presentations

- Conduct patient safety rounds

- Cultivate patient satisfaction

- Relentlessly focus on operations

- Build reliability into your system

Military aviation and urgent care medicine

Establishing a culture of safety in the aviation industry has been a core focus for many years. In fact, many safety techniques that other industries have adopted come from aviation. Military aviation, in particular, has a significant connection to urgent care medicine. Studies of crashes and near misses in the military revealed that the single biggest cause of accidents was miscommunication. In response, the military developed crew resource management (CRM), a training methodology that focuses on teaching team members to work

---

together as a coordinated unit. This type of training greatly reduced the number of crashes.

The teamwork connection

Dynamics Research Corporation (DRC), which was involved in the military development of CRM, and other organizations adopted the principles of CRM and implemented these methods in urgent care medicine. DRC's MedTeams program is one example of that approach, which not only improves quality of care, but also enhances patient safety. Teamwork skills, particularly situational awareness, are central in establishing a culture of safety. A technique that helps reinforce situational awareness is the SBAR tool: situation, background, assessment, and recommendation. Team members can use this tool in communicating with each other regarding a patient. The following description shows how:

- Situation = Describing the situation with clear facts and figures (e.g., pulse rate, respiration, and concerns)

- Background = Describing the patient's background

- Assessment = Giving a clear assessment of the problem

- Recommendations = Making recommendations on managing the case

This process may seem simple, but having an established protocol like this can help healthcare organizations build a culture of safety with team members communicating effectively in your urgent care center.

Reviewing actions

As we observed earlier, healthcare professionals do not come to work intending to make mistakes. Studies of errors in many industries show that initial blame for 70% to 80% of errors falls on the last person involved in the situation. Subsequent investigation, however, usually finds that the last person involved actually accounts for less than 20% of the error. After-action reviews provide a method to examine what went wrong in the system when a mistake happens.

Charles Vincent et al. found that reviews of accidents' causes should focus less on the individual who makes the error and more on preexisting organizational factors because of the complex chain of events that may lead to an adverse outcome.[4] Ultimate causes of errors may include excessive workload and training deficiencies, for example.

When you conduct an after-action review, ask the following questions:

- What were the intended results and how were we going to measure them?

- What challenges should we have anticipated in this case?

- What have we or others learned from similar situations?

- What will enable us to succeed in a similar case?

By talking with all of the key people involved, you can learn about the case sequentially and fine-tune what questions to ask in follow-up discussions. After you talk to all people involved, go back and talk to the first people you spoke with, armed with your acquired knowledge about the events surrounding the case.

Catching the Errors

Traditionally, patient safety models created an underlying atmosphere of fear by focusing on who was at fault rather than focusing on processes. This type of environment and fear of punishment drives errors underground. Errors are not reported, and no one can learn from them, leaving the system unchanged and the errors recurring.

In order to learn from errors and near misses and create a safer, more effective urgent care center, you should take a fundamentally different approach by establishing a nonpunitive model. Drive out fear. Your staff members must believe reporting errors is a high priority of your operation and it will not get them in trouble.

Figure 11.1 provides one way to help achieve this goal. The error report chart helps encourage team members to turn in near misses and mistakes. It is simple to create and provides an effective way to learn what is happening in your urgent care center. Use it for three months to track the categories listed in the figure, and then examine the patterns.

FIGURE 11.1

AN ERROR-REPORT CHART

INCIDENT	RECORD NUMBER	TYPE	SUGGESTIONS FOR IMPROVEMENT	RESULTS

Managing risk

If you know who's going to come to your urgent care center and why they're coming, then you can prepare to handle high-risk situations. Take the top 10 to 20 closed malpractice cases with the greatest prevalence for urgent care physicians and establish best practices for treating these types of cases (see Figure 11.2).

For example, how should urgent care centers handle a patient with testicular torsion? The best practice for patients with an acute onset of testicular pain and a clinical finding of torsion is the following:

- An immediate call to the urologist

- Attempted manual detorsion

- Immediate surgery as definitive treatment

FIGURE 11.2

TOP 10 DIAGNOSES INVOLVED IN ED CLAIMS, BY TOTAL NUMBER OF CLOSED CLAIMS

Acute myocardial infarction
Chest pain, not further defined
Symptoms involving abdomen and pelvis
Injury to multiple parts of the body
Appendicitis
Fracture of vertebral column
Fracture of radius or ulna
Aortic aneurysm
Open wound to fingers
Fracture of the tibia or fibula

Source: ACADEMIC EMERGENCY MEDICINE 2010: 17:553-560 © 2012 by the Society for Academic Emergency Medicine

---

Every patient with testicular torsion as a presumptive diagnosis should get an ultrasound and a urological consultation, or be referred to an emergency department (ED). Following this procedure as standard practice allows you to clinically rule in testicular torsion definitively. If the procedure is embedded into your urgent care practice, the urgent care physicians and nurses know it.

Following this approach at Best Practices allowed us to reduce this serious condition by 70% in one year. One result among several positive ones was a decrease in malpractice insurance premiums. In addition, satisfaction increased among physicians, nurses, and patients. Standardizing an evidence-based format for the other closed-case malpractice experiences enables you to manage risk in these situations effectively and reduce risk significantly.

Safety rounds

Clinic leaders should conduct regular safety rounds throughout the center, both to see for themselves how operations are proceeding and how the urgent care center looks and to ask staff members (and perhaps patients as well) questions to learn where the center can improve. Leaders should ask themselves the following types of questions:

- Is the center clean?

- Are the processes working effectively?

- Is it clinically safe?

Allan Frankel and colleagues developed an initiative for the Institute for Healthcare Improvement, known as WalkRounds, which lays out in detail a process for conducting this type of rounds.[5] It enables administrators and various staff members to discuss safety conditions in the center confidentially. Under this process, leaders routinely ask the following questions to elicit information from staff members:

- Have there been any near misses?

- Have there been any incidents recently that concern you or your team members?

- What can we do to prevent an adverse event?

Once you have established a blame-free culture for error reporting, these conversations can provide valuable feedback from the clinicians doing the work on the urgent care center floor.

Frankel et al. also describe how information gathered in these rounds can be entered into a tracking database and then categorized by contributing factors. This process assigns a score to the event based on potential impact and frequency. Tracking and analyzing data in this way helps you respond effectively to safety issues.

Patient satisfaction

Patient satisfaction and patient safety go hand in hand; when patients are satisfied, usually that means conditions are safer, and vice versa. We mentioned checking to see if your urgent care facility is clean, for example. A clean center is a safer one, and it will make patients more content about being there.

As in many other aspects of urgent care operations, effective communication leads to more satisfied patients. Consider one study that found, for example, that 71% of patients who sued for malpractice cited a poor relationship with staff as the reason for their legal action. Of those patients, 32% felt deserted and 29% felt devalued.[6] Good communication reduces the risk of malpractice litigation. It also inherently makes the urgent care center safer.

How your center handles complaints should be as important as preventing them. The center's clinicians should follow a protocol for resolving patient complaints with timely and detailed personal contact with the patient involved. Take advantage of the opportunity to gather data you can track and analyze for trends. Circulate the results of this analysis with all clinicians in the center to improve performance.

Stay Focused on Ongoing Operations

The man with insight enough to admit his limitations comes nearest to perfection.

—Johann von Goethe

By tracking and analyzing data and testing changes, you are reducing complexity, improving communication, and decreasing the likelihood of error. The more you can monitor operations, examine what is happening, and adjust the processes, the more you can prevent mistakes. We've emphasized how to deal with errors, but don't lose sight of how much more effective and safer you can make your urgent care center by preventing them.

Coaching should be an important part of your effort to stay focused on operations as well. To reduce risk, organize diagnostic categories for high-risk conditions. Provide education on a common approach to these conditions to physicians, midlevel providers, and nurses. Use white papers and PowerPoint® presentations to outline evaluation, diagnosis, and treatment for each category. Then follow up with competency quizzes to test how well your team has absorbed the educational material. You want to increase both competency and accountability.

This type of an educational program should have a pediatric and adult components. The adult module should address the 10 conditions listed in the section on managing risk. Figure 11.3 shows what categories the pediatric module should include.

The urgent care clinic should require new clinicians to complete these modules within a prescribed time; we recommend 90 days. Some group practices also require annual or biannual recertification to be eligible for certain bonuses. This process heightens participation on a team, creates a common language for

---

FIGURE 11.3
COMMON PEDIATRIC CONDITIONS

Pediatric fever
Abdominal pain
Head injury
Orthopedic injuries (growth plate)
Wound care (both adult and pediatric)
Asthma
Child abuse

---

clinicians and nursing staff, and supports a learning environment to enable your staff to better understand certain clinical cases and allow them to intervene thoroughly and predictably. The more you simplify decision-making, the more you increase effectiveness and reduce risk.

Building a reliable system

Reliability comes from emphasizing the following factors:

- Standardizing processes

- Introducing redundancy

- Identifying critical failures

- Redesigning processes

The following example from everyday life demonstrates how to build reliability into your processes. In the past when you have used an automated teller machine (ATM), you put in your card and it gave you your money. Then you pushed a button to get your card back. Predictably, many individuals forgot to retrieve their cards, causing worry and work for both customer and the bank. Finally, banks examined the process and redesigned it. With newer ATMs, you must take your card back before the machine dispenses your cash. The redesign built safety and reliability into the ATM system.

Follow-up care

Standardizing processes and introducing redundancy is important for patient follow-up issues. The most common areas of error with follow-up involve testing.

It is critical for urgent care centers to develop failsafe processes to ensure that final test results are documented, acted upon, and communicated to the patient. The three most common areas of testing error are the following:

- Completing culture results (e.g. urine, throat, etc.)

- Sending out lab tests

- Reading final x-ray results

Failure to provide closure with these issues may result in patient harm, adverse outcome, and litigation. Consider the following processes to ensure no harm occurs.

Culture results

1. Designate a single person to be responsible for tracking down all culture results on a daily basis

2. Consider developing a culture log to ease the process

3. Develop a simple form for positive culture results identifying the patient, the results, and a space to document any changes in therapy required

4. Present all culture results to the attending physician (preferably earlier in the morning when there are limited distractions), ensure that the attending physician completes the form

5. Require the physician to sign the results

6.   The person in step No. 1 (or the physicians) makes contact with the patient informing them of the results and any needed changes in therapy.

7.   File the results in the patient's chart. (Ensure that all staff understands that no results are filed in the chart unless a visible, legible physician signature is present.)

Sending out tests

This is often required for prostate-specific antigen (PSA) tests, complex tests, but may also include CBC and comprehensive metabolic panels when the site only has waive testing.

1.   Designate a single person to be responsible for tracking down all send-out tests on a daily basis.

2.   Have a process that all patient charts with any send-out lab requests are placed in a "holding bend" to ensure that when tests are returned they can be addressed. In addition, charts remaining in the holding bend can be pulled and reviewed to determine why the results have not returned.

3.   Develop a simple form for test results identifying the patient, the results, and a space to document any changes in therapy required.

4.   Present all test results to the attending physician (preferably earlier in the morning when there are limited distractions), ensure that the attending physician completes the form.

5.   Require the physician to sign the results.

6.   The person in step No. 1 (or the physicians) makes contact with the patient informing them of the results and any needed changes in therapy.

7.   File the results in the patient's chart. (Ensure that all staff understands that no results are filed in the chart unless a visible, legible physician signature is present.)

Radiology discrepancy

Some clinics will have x-rays taken and perform the initial read by the attending physician on-site. This often occurs during after hours and weekend patient visits. These films have a final interpretation completed by the radiologist (we recommend this in all cases; one missed chest mass/malignancy will result in patient harm and major litigation costs).

1.   You should have a predeveloped process and list of "critical findings" (collapsed lung, etc.) that are directly called by the radiologist to the attending physician at the clinic immediately.

2.   Develop a process where the initial reading of the x-ray is documented by the attending physician and can been seen by the radiologist. The radiologist can then determine if there was a discrepancy and contact the site directly.

3.   Consider having all final radiology readings print out on a specific computer at a specific time each day. These results can then be reviewed comparing initial reading with final to ensure correct interpretation.

4.   Present any discrepancies to the attending physician (it does not matter how trivial the discrepancy; a "small" density on a chest film can become a big deal).

5.   Follow the same pattern as above.

We can apply similar principles in medicine. The following is an example, dealing with community-acquired pneumonia. Triage in an urgent care center that is intent on building reliability has established triggers when someone over 50 years of age arrives with a productive cough, high temperature, and other symptoms suggestive of pneumonia. The triage staff automatically flags that patient for a chest x-ray. Once the physician or midlevel provider makes a diagnosis of pneumonia, another trigger alerts the pharmacy, which then automatically sends a message back to the urgent care center: "Is this patient on the pneumonia pathway?" If the x-ray indicates pneumonia, the radiology center has a trigger in its system that flags pneumonia for the urgent care center and then asks if the patient is being treated accordingly. Figure 11.4 diagrams how this type of process would flow.

Urgent care centers should standardize information, reporting forms, and procedures to reduce variation. If the layout of your center separates work groups or disrupts processes, then redesign it to smooth actual physical flow within it. Group types of work with similar requirements, and automate repetitive operations.

FIGURE 11.4

COMMUNITY-ACQUIRED PNEUMONIA PROTOCOL MODEL FOR THE URGENT CARE CENTER

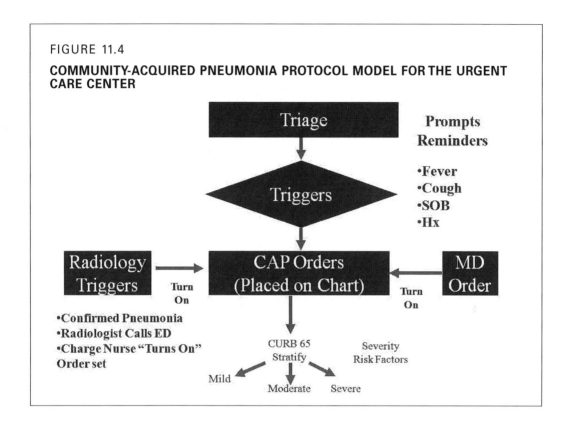

Building reliability into your system will enable you to go from one error in every 10 cases to one error in every 100. When you achieve that goal, you will have greatly improved the quality of your care and the safety of your environment.

REFERENCES

1. Leape, Lucien. Error in Medicine. JAMA. 1994. 272(23): 1851-1857.

2. Vincent, Charles, et al. Framework for Analyzing Risk and Safety in Clinical Medicine. BJM. 1998. 316(7138): 1154-1157.

3. Nolan, T.W. System Changes to Improve Patient Safety. BMJ. 2000. 320: 771-773.

4. ibid.

5. Frankel, Allan, et al. Revealing and Resolving Patient Safety Defects: The Impact of Leadership WalkRounds on Frontline Caregiver Assessments of Patient Safety. Health Serv Res. 2008 December; 43(6): 2050–2066.

6. Beckman, H.B., et al. The Doctor-Patient Relationship and Malpractice: Lessons from Plaintiff's Depositions. Archives of Internal Medicine. 1994. 154(12): 1365.

Strategies to Expand Urgent Care Business

In addition to injury and illness care, urgent care centers are ideal sites to provide programs in occupational medicine, physical examination (e.g., sports, school, camp, executives, and immigrants), immunization, and travel medicine. In addition, hospital-affiliated urgent care centers provide a relief valve for the emergency department (ED) by providing afterhours access for patients of medical staff members, follow-up care for patients from the ED and hospital postdischarge, among others. The following are common questions asked about expanding an urgent care center's business model from the traditional minor illness and injury service.

- What programs can be developed to supplement urgent care volume?

- How should an occupational medicine program be structured?

- What types of physical examinations should the clinic offer and are there risks?

- What are developing new trends offered by urgent care facilities?

- As part of a hospital system, what role can the urgent care center play in the system?

BUSINESS EXPANSION DEFINITIONS

Civil surgeon: A medical professional that has completed the requirements developed by U.S. Citizenship and Immigrations Services for the performance of required physical examinations on all immigrants requesting any change in the status of their visa or citizenship application.

Medical review officer (MRO): This is a physician that has undergone specialized training in the evaluation, interpretation, and follow-up of employee drug screens. They typically are certified by a state program as qualified to review drug screens. Drug screens may be required by employers in a random fashion or after injury/accident. Negative-result drug screens are simple and straightforward. The collection methodology, however, and false negative results (patients dilute urine or use someone else's urine specimen) are nuances that a trained MRO can detect. The difficulty lies in determining whether a positive drug screen is truly positive (e.g., poppy seeds causing a false positive opiate screen) and what steps need to be taken to protect both the employee and employer with positive screens. This presents liability to the MRO, the employee, and the employer when a screen (negative, positive, or equivocal) is handled inappropriately.

Occupational medicine marketer: This is the person who presents the offered product to the employers, sets up specific protocols for employees, sets up referral panels for employees, and becomes the voice of the site to the employer. They should be responsible for program development and continued growth.

Company profile: These are guidelines set up for each contracted company. Items that are critical include a specific referral panel for specialty care (orthopedics, etc.), requirements of postaccident drug screening, specification regarding light duty/return to work, and identification of postinjury follow-up.

Occupational Medicine

Since the beginning of the urgent care medical model, occupational medicine practice has developed into a natural outgrowth of urgent care. Urgent care centers often provide preemployment physicals, random and postinjury drug screening, and injury management. This review is merely provided as a brief overview of program development.

Employers seek clinics that treat their employees quickly, provide appropriate care and specialty referral (within the company panel), provide follow-up care at competitive costs, and return injured employees back to work as soon as possible. Occupational medicine relies on established relationships with employers and access for employees to both afterhours and follow-up care.

Worker's compensation has become very onerous due to paperwork, referral approvals, a lack of participating specialist providers in state programs, return-to-work issues, medical and legal issues, among others. The majority of primary care physicians actually avoids these patients, because of the challenging nature of offering occupational medicine services. The clinical spectrum of care for occupational medicine matches that of urgent care with some add-on services, such as physical examinations and specialized testing. At one of our sites in New York, we became the provider by default, because the ED could find no follow-up care for these patients.

Physicals

Physical examinations are a major component of occupational medicine and often provide an easy revenue source for the clinic, but this service should be done with care to avoid potential liability. Marketing to municipal organizations, including fire departments, police, local schools, etc., is a very good source for contracting. For instance, pulmonary function testing and audiometry are often components of firefighter evaluation and would require the appropriate equipment for performance of these specific exams.

Similarly, Department of Transportation (DOT) and Federal Aviation Administration (FAA) physicals are unique subsets for physical exams performed on bus drivers, truckers, and pilots, among others. Any driver operating vehicles that transport passengers or property between states is required to have Federal Medical Certification by the Federal Motor Carrier Administration (FMCSA).[1] The FMCSA also maintains a national registry of certified medical examiners. To become certified, the applicant must complete a course and pass an examination. Information on the course and examination are available at *http://nrcme.fmcsa .dot.gov*. There are manuals explicitly describing the entire process, including requirements for hearing, vision, current medical conditions, medications, and components of the complete physical examination. Information for the DOT exam process and the DOT physical examination manual providing information for medical providers can be found at *www.fmcsa.dot.gov/rules-regulations/ topics/medical/aboutdotexam.htm*. In addition, Federal Aviation Administration exam information can be found at *www.faa.gov/about/office_org/headquarters_ offices/avs/offices/aam/ame/guide/app_process/exam_tech*. FAA and DOT physicals can provide a revenue stream of $150 to $250 per physical.[2] The goals of these examinations are to ensure that the examinee has no significant medical condition that could result in or contribute to the cause of a vehicle or airplane accident, thereby potentially excluding the examined patient from commercial driving or piloting of an aircraft.

Care protocols

The most common injuries involve skin and soft tissue (e.g., lacerations, abrasions); musculoskeletal overuse, such as strain of neck or back; fractures; hand and wrist injuries (e.g., sprain, carpel tunnel, fracture, tendinitis, tendon laceration or rupture); knee injuries (e.g., sprain, meniscal tear, ligament tear); and ankle and foot injuries (e.g., sprain and ligament tear, especially Achilles and ankle collaterals). Excluding fractures, many state worker compensation programs and insurance carriers have developed a well-defined algorithm to follow for each area. Treatment for these services often follow a standard protocol, including the initial injury that was seen in the ED and referred to the clinic, follow-up care, diagnostics testing, followed by specialty referral or return to work. The program in New York (*www.wcb.ny.gov*) provides step-by-step guidelines for care, and following those guidelines will significantly improve reimbursement from the program.

For example, a patient injured his back with a twisting mechanism and presented to the ED. Conservative care is elected, and the patient in referred to an urgent care clinic for follow up in one to two days. When the patient arrives at the clinics, symptoms have not improved, and medication is continued or instituted with a scheduled follow-up visit. The plan of care dictates tests recommended with deviations that can occur, but only with appropriate indication and documentation. For example, if the patient has back pain but no neurologic deficits, and an MRI is ordered, the exam may not be paid for because it did not follow the treatment pathway or include a reason for deviation from the treatment pathway. These pathways have been well researched and validated, and adherence to these protocols is often tied to reimbursement for both care and testing.

Panel

Your center should maintain a referral schedule for specific injuries, including hand surgery (e.g., tendon repair and hand fractures), orthopedic surgery for fractures in general, physical therapy (it is preferable to have the same institution provide physical therapy), ophthalmology (e.g., corneal abrasion and corneal foreign body removal), neurology (e.g., complicated head injury, concussive syndromes, and neuropathy evaluation, including carpel tunnel and nerve conduction studies), and neurosurgery (e.g., disc herniation refractory to conservative care and physical therapy). Other specialties may be needed depending on the injury and the employer preference. The employer may already have a referral program that should be included in the employer-specific profile, or the facility can provide a preferred profile. The specialist relationship with a clinic's preferred profile must include accountability with assured same-day or next-day appointment and communication with the clinic. Failure to provide this service to the clinic should result in elimination of that specialist from the referral panel.

Drug screening

Companies frequently require drug screening in a random fashion and postinjury. Urgent care clinics provide these services, which contribute additional revenue to the clinic and the laboratory, especially if the lab is owned or affiliated with the clinic. Drug screening requires understanding the collection process and methods to detect fraudulent samples (e.g., using another person's urine, diluting urine samples, and using adulterants to result in false-negative results). In addition, the clinic's restroom facilities (toilets) need to be set up in an appropriate manner to avoid specimen tampering. Physicians reviewing the drug screen must have certification that requires periodic renewal. Most drug screens are negative and are simple to interpret by the medical review officer. It is the positive drug screen that requires careful handling. The medical review officer (MRO) must ensure that the screen is a true positive rather than a false positive (e.g., a positive opiate screen after the ingestion of poppy seeds). Ensuring the sample was interpreted correctly protects the employee from and clinic from inappropriate disciplinary actions and legal challenges, respectively.

Finally, occupational medicine follow-up exams and postinjury evaluation and physical exams can be scheduled during times of low clinic volume to maximize clinic utilization and revenue. Many states and insurance carriers, however, provide limited reimbursement for postinjury follow-up care. In our experience, this reimbursement often ranges between $30 and $40 dollars per visit. This may also be a bundled reimbursement, which means this "global fee" covers the entire costs for both the professional component and clinic fee. You should ensure that your cost structure and clinic efficiency allow for these lower levels of reimbursement. Combining paperwork requirements, state certification, and challenges with referrals, clinics must weigh carefully the risk and benefit of a full-service occupational medicine program.

Marketing (occupational medicine)

A key component of any occupational medicine program is promoting the urgent care clinic's services to increase its occupational medicine business along with injury evaluation and follow-up. The designated marketer should meet with company safety officers, employee health nurses, and administrators when selling the program; maintain the relationship; and assist in resolving problems that arise between the clinic, employee, and the company. They should work with each company in the development of specific corporate profiles to be available in the clinic that define requirements for postinjury drug screening, specialty referral panels, and availability of light duty for injured workers, etc.

Immunization Clinic

As part of an accountable care organization, urgent care centers would play a vital role in patient access, allowing for disease prevention. Immunizations are a key component in disease prevention. It does not take a long memory to recall the pandemic of 2009, with overcrowding of influenza patients in EDs, clinics, and physician offices. Many patients were simply turned away from private physician offices and referred to EDs, because physician offices couldn't handle the volume of patients. The 2010 and 2011 influenza seasons were much less dramatic, and we would like to believe that immunizations were a primary reason for this. Your center may have, as part of its mission statement, a goal to prevent disease and promote health. Immunization programs do just that.

Figure 12.1 suggests the approximate costs and charges that are used for immunizations at one of our sites. Obviously, costs will vary by quantity and

FIGURE 12.1

URGENT CARE IMMUNIZATION COSTS/CHARGES *

	COST	CHARGE	COMMENTS
Influenza	$9.64	$28.56	pts > 3 years old
Hepatitis A			
#1	$54.22	$162.69	per dose charge
#2	$54.22	$162.69	per dose charge
Hepatitis B			
#1	$18.17	$54.52	per dose charge
#2	$18.17	$54.52	per dose charge
#3	$18.17	$52.52	per dose charge
Meningococcal	$104.37	$313.11	
Pneumococcal	$52.52	$157.57	
Td	$16.51	$49.53	
Tdap	$30.06	$90.17	indicated for pts age 11–64
Herpes Zoster	$160.00	$480.00	
HPV	$120.52	$361.56	
Tb test	$2.09	$8.72	per test charge

*These figures are only estimates. There is potential for add on charges for the nursing injection codes per-
formed by the nursing staff member.

pharmaceutical contracts, and charges differ by system charge schedules. In addition, the urgent care site may charge an injection fee that typically is between $10 and $25. Immunization services can be marketed, but each must include patient education, indications, and contraindications for use, followed by consent from the patient for injection. Many insurance programs, including Medicaid and Medicare, cover the majority of the immunizations listed in Figure 12.2.

> ## BUSINESS EXPANSION DEFINITIONS
>
> **Civil surgeon:** A medical professional that has completed the requirements developed by U.S. Citizenship and Immigrations Services for the performance of required physical examinations on all immigrants requesting any change in the status of their visa or citizenship application.
>
> **Medical review officer (MRO):** This is a physician that has undergone specialized training in the evaluation, interpretation, and follow-up of employee drug screens. They

Marketing discounts for specific immunizations may increase business; this strategy is often used by retail pharmacies.

Travel Medicine

International travel has become quite popular, and many travelers require education, immunizations, and medication prophylaxis. Combining an immunization clinic with medical travel consulting, the clinic provides patients with a full-service product. Expansion into travel medicine requires that providers become proficient in the service by obtaining both education and certification in the specialty before providing detailed advice and care to travelers. Travel clinics provide a pretravel assessment; evaluate the traveler's health status and potential risks for travel, such as deep vein thrombosis (DVT) prevention; provide needed immunizations for travel to the specified area, education on the availability of healthcare in the region being traveled to, education on local food and water preparation, and information about precautions and prophylaxis for potential disease exposures, including malaria.

The pretravel assessment should be a planned appointment where the patient brings a complete immunization record for review, medication list, travel itinerary, medical history, and type of travel planned. Screening the patient's medical history and medications assist in recommendations, such as ensuring the patient has ample medication for the trip and additional doses in the event of trip delay. In addition, plans can be made for medication loss and replacement by knowing the region of travel. This reduces the likelihood of the patient foregoing critical medication, such as insulin. It is also critical to address the need for international health insurance along with emergency evacuation insurance in the event that these are required. Travelers should also consider dental visits before departure to ensure issues are addressed rather than requiring dental care in a foreign nation or having the pain ruin a vacation. Education regarding personal safety, international driving, and crime may also help prevent injury. Educating travelers regarding DVT prevention; infectious disease exposures, including blood-borne illness (e.g., hepatitis and HIV); and sexually transmitted disease prevention is critical.

The location and type of travel affect the counseling and potential medication prophylaxis significantly. There is a major difference in travel to Costa Rica or other areas of Central America on board a cruise ship and hiking through the rain forest for days. The former is unlikely to require antimalarial medication but may require medication for motion sickness. The latter may need insect-born repellent such as DEET (*N*,*N*-dimethyl-meta-toluamide) or picaridin to reduce mosquito exposure and disease. Applying repellents to clothing the day before use, along with the use of bed netting, also reduces exposure. Finally, the need for antimalarial prophylaxis is determined based on region of travel. It is imperative that the clinic ensures that

---

medication interaction with antimalarials is addressed before you provide the medication.

Food and water consumption in foreign countries often leads to water-borne illness, especially in lesser-developed countries. These areas may have potential for hepatitis A exposure that requires vaccination. Also, food hygiene includes avoiding street vendors, salads, and uncooked or undercooked meats/seafood; drinking boiled or bottled water; avoiding ice; and avoiding unpasteurized dairy products.[3]

Immunizations are a critical component of travel medicine. Many countries require documentation with an immunization record (e.g., International Certificate of Vaccination or Prophylaxis [IVCP]), especially countries with yellow fever risk. They require a specific stamp certifying that immunization has been done. Yellow fever immunizations require certification of a provider through the state. More common immunizations include hepatitis A and B, tetanus (Td or Tdap), MMR (measles, mumps, rubella), influenza, and pneumococcal. For travelers unsure of immunizations, serologic tests are available for hepatitis A and B, measles, and varicella, rather than repeating the vaccination.

For high-adventure travelers, education and medication for high-altitude illness may be required along with information regarding the safety and timing of air travel after SCUBA diving. There is information regarding travel medicine through the Centers for Disease Control and Prevention (CDC), and information is available through the government at *www.nc.cdc.gov/travel/*. In addition, the urgent care clinic would benefit from the experience of an available infectious disease consultant. Although there are abundant resources and guidelines provided by the Infectious Disease Society of America and CDC, providers should consider specialized training and certification before providing more than the basic travel medicine counseling and consulting, as suggested before.[4]

Physical Examinations

Access to primary care physicians—even for patients with insurance—can be challenging aside from scheduling routine physical examinations. Urgent care centers and retail clinics help fill this void by providing physical examinations for school, sports, camps, immigration, and executives. The purpose of these examinations is to determine whether the person is medically fit to perform or participate in a specific task. DOT, FAA, and immigration examinations are performed to protect the public as a method of accident prevention in DOT/FAA and public exposure reduction (e.g., tuberculosis) for immigration physicals. Obviously, revenue is generated from the physical exam itself, but ancillary testing, immunizations, and imaging procedures add to the full package.

Sports and school physicals are excellent public relations and marketing tools. In addition, clinic or healthcare systems could also ensure that the athletic venues are equipped with automatic external defibrillators (AED) and educational programs for coaches regarding head trauma and heat illness prevention during summer practices.

School

Most school athletic programs require a complete physical exam and physician/healthcare provider release prior to participation. These often require only 15 to

30 minutes, with charge in the $50 range per physical. Unfortunately, within the thousands of young healthy students, there are some with significant risk for disease and death related to sporting activity. Football and basketball have the highest risk of sudden death in the United States, whereas soccer has the highest risk in the rest of the world.[5] This subset of the population highlights the risks any sports physical program should understand and manage by appropriate specialty referrals. Each clinic should weigh the financial benefit of sports physicals with the risk of a single missed high-risk athlete and bad outcome.[6]

One caution for examiners is the high-risk participant, including athletes with heart murmurs, chest pain, or a history of exercise-induced syncope. Hypertrophic cardiomyopathy is a leading cause of death in athletes that is difficult to detect on routine physical exam, along with other causes listed in Figure 12.3.[7,8] You should consider referral to a cardiologist for evaluation of cardiac structural abnormalities with an echocardiogram and exertion-related arrhythmia with stress testing (see Figure 12.4). In addition, athletes (and their parents) with both recent and remote head injury from contact sports should be educated on repetitive concussions and the risk to health and learning. Both of these categories, cardiac and neurologic, may be sources of malpractice risk for the provider if not handled appropriately.

Camp/school/college

Like the above-described exams, camp, school, and college physicals are similar and may be charged at a similar level. Most require only a simple physical exam; however, some may require basic lab testing. To improve efficiency, a standard

FIGURE 12.3

SUDDEN CAUSE OF DEATH IN AN ATHLETE

Sudden cardiac death
- Hypertrophic cardiomyopathy
- Anomalous coronary arteries
- Myocarditis
- Arrhythmias (ion channel disorders, WPW, Bruguda syndrome)
- Commotio cordis
- Aortic stenosis

Other
- Exercise-induced asthma
- Head trauma

FIGURE 12.4

RED FLAGS FOR SPECIALTY REFERRAL

History
- Sudden death in a family member under the age of 50 and death of unknown cause in a family member
- Family history of Marfan's syndrome, cardiac disease at a young age
- Chest pain (especially exertional)
- Palpitations
- Exertional dyspnea (other than deconditioning)
- Syncope/presyncope (especially exertional, but any episode should raise concern)

Exam
- Hypertension
- Cardiac murmur
- Unequal radial versus femoral pulses
- Irregular pulses

template can assist the urgent care medical provider in rapid completion of required documentation for a complete physical examination.

Immigration

Immigrants applying for citizenship, work visas, or adjustments in his or her residency status are required to undergo an immigration physical.[9] These exams can be performed only by physicians designated in the U.S. Citizenship and Immigrations Services (USCIS) and certified as a Civil Surgeon (CS). CS positions may be applied for through the regional USCIS office and are limited in number based on region. After application completion and approval, the CS becomes a listed provider on the USCIS website. Much of the work for these programs involves gathering and completing paperwork. Training office personnel to gather required information and developing templates or checklists allows for a smoother operation and improved efficiency of the CS. Syphilis testing is required; therefore, affiliation with a reference lab is needed. Similar to DOT and FAA physicals, the examination requirements are provided in detail from the USCIS along with the certifying process at *www.uscis.gov*. These exams may be charged at a level similar to that of an extensive physical ($100–$200) in addition to any required immunizations or ancillary testing. This program is especially beneficial in cities having a higher level of immigration and international workers and students.

Executive

Executive management of large and small corporations is essential for business success. Loss of an executive, especially the CEO, can be a financial challenge or even economic tragedy for any company. The health of the executive is critical, and health maintenance, including a complete physical exam, is essential. This examination should be thorough, with extensive laboratory profiles, including evaluation of lipids, PSA (for males), cardiac risk panels/CRP, comprehensive metabolic panels, etc. Each exam may require up to one full hour and should be charged as such. In addition to the complete physical examination, considerations should include exercise stress testing to assist in detecting early cardiac disease. Other tests could include cardiac computed tomography evaluating cardiac risk and abdominal scanning (ultrasound or CAT scanning) to evaluate for an aneurysm. The provider should determine the benefits for these tests based on need compared to the risk of unnecessary radiation exposure. Companies will readily pay for these exams as an insurance policy for early detection or disease prevention. Finally, all patients should be counseled for smoking cessation, reduced alcohol consumption, and healthy lifestyles.

Hospital-Affiliated Clinics

Hospital-affiliated clinics can provide several services that result in significant benefit to the organization. The urgent care clinic can be used for referral from the ED for lower-acuity patients screened out of the ED. In addition, it is often difficult to get close follow-up care for patients with simple wound rechecks, hypertension reevaluation, suture removals, cellulitis, and many others. This becomes especially critical when patients lack a primary care physician. In addition, follow-up care acts to decongest the ED along with follow-up in a more cost-effective and appropriate environment.

For the hospital medical staff, the clinic provides afterhours accessibility for staff members. This function is especially helpful with a completely integrated electronic medical record, providing the medical staff member with immediate information and results from the patient visit. The clinic can provide postdischarge follow-up for patients with congestive heart failure, chronic obstructive pulmonary disease, and cellulitis in an attempt to reduce hospital readmission. Finally, we have seen many disasters cause the closure of hospital emergency departments or result in overwhelming volume. Hospital-affiliated urgent care centers may be a partial solution when disasters strikes a healthcare facility by providing an alternative treatment site—especially when combined with an adjacent imaging center.

REFERENCES

1. Wittels, E. 2010. Providing the DOT Medical Certification Exams for Commercial Drivers. J Urgent Care Med. September:13–20.

2. Boyle, M. 2011. Tap into new revenue streams. Medical Economics. 88(15):24–25, 31–32, 35.

3. Olmstead, F. 2010. The Traveling Patient. 2010. J Urgent Care Med. February:11.

4. Hill, D., Ericsson C., et al. 2006. The Practice of Travel Medicine: Guidelines by the Infectious Disease Society of America. Clin Infect Dis. 43:1499–1539.

5. Ibid.

6. Shufeldt, J. 2011. Are Urgent Care Liable. J Urgent Care Med. September:29–30.

7. Ibid.

8. Newman, N. 2011. Sudden Cardiac Death: Identifying Risk Factors in Participation Physicals for Young Athletes. J Urgent Care Med. September:9–19.

9. Ayers, A. 2011. Enhancing Profits with Immigration Physicals. J Urgent Care Med. May:23–29.

The Freestanding Emergency Department

The concept of freestanding emergency departments (FED) was developed during the late 1970s, with one of the first being ACCESS of Reston, which is affiliated with the Inova Health System in Fairfax, Va. FED sites are larger than urgent care centers, have longer hours of operation, and have greater service capability.

When you consider developing a FED, you need an understanding of state and federal guidelines. Most FED sites are hospital affiliated, but several private facilities have emerged. The unique challenge these sites face occurs with disposition of patients requiring admission or specialty care.

Principles of the Freestanding Emergency Department

The Centers for Medicare and Medicaid Services (CMS) has categorized FEDs into the following two types:

- Type A: Licensed by the state, advertised to the public as providing emergency services, open 24 hours per day, seven days per week

- Type B: Dedicated emergency department (ED) operating less than 24 hours per day

We define FEDs as sites that are open 24 hours per day, seven days per week; maintain full lab capability (other than extensive microbiology processes); provide basic radiology, ultrasound, and CT scanning; and accept ambulance transfers. Staffing includes emergency physicians, certified nurses, and technicians. Most sites are hospital owned, with approximately 241 facilities as of 2009 in 16 states.

Design

Many FEDs are built to provide a health system with a footprint in new areas or capture patients from competing organizations. The size of FEDs is far larger than urgent care centers. They are well over 10,000 square feet and require space for lab, radiology, and usually 10 or more treatment rooms.

For hospital-owned facilities, state and local code requirements are much more stringent regarding patient care room sizes, the need for a clean and soiled utility, and specifications for lab and radiology spaces. The American College of Emergency Physicians' "Emergency Department Design: A Practical Guide to Planning for the Future" is an excellent resource for space requirements and design basics.[1] In addition, the American Institute of Architects (AIA) publishes "Guidelines for Design and Construction of Hospital and Health Care Facilities," which is also an excellent reference.

As we mentioned in Chapter 4, a qualified medical architect is of immense value in helping administrators determining their needs and meeting regulatory requirements.

Equipment and supplies

The supplies and equipment needed for FEDs are similar to the equipment list for urgent care centers that is found in Appendix A. Most beds will need to be a stretcher tip for mobility purposes rather than the short examination table. In addition, FEDs require additional resuscitation equipment for adult and pediatric patients and an expanded medication list, including a larger list of cardiac and antibiotic medications.

Administrators will need to determine if they need high-dollar thrombolytic drugs that have expiration dates and may become an inventory cost concern. That decision will depend on the distance and time requirements to transfer for acute myocardial infarction and stroke patients. In addition, several beds require cardiac, pulse oximetry, and end tidal CO_2 monitoring. Finally, the site requires all modalities of airway management, including advanced airway equipment inclusive of surgical and fiberoptic options. It is unlikely the FED has access to an anesthesiologist as most hospital-based EDs have; therefore, all adjunctive airways modalities should be available.

Licensing

State licensing requirements vary considerably in regard to FEDs. Rhode Island was the first state to develop regulations for FEDs.[2] Illinois has developed specific licensing for FEDs, whereas Texas does not consider them components of the hospital and only recently developed licensing guidelines. Florida (and many other states) requires a certificate of need (CON) and placed a moratorium on FEDs that expired in 2006.[3] CON programs apply to healthcare systems and hospitals, with less influence on independent physicians.[4]

Legislation is rapidly changing regarding FEDs, and it is crucial to be up to date on your state's specific requirements. CMS, on the other hand, has opened acceptance to FEDs and requires them to be organized and supervised by a qualified medical staff member, be integrated with other hospital departments, governed by medical staff–approved policies, and furnish adequate numbers of qualified medical personnel.[5] One distinct component of an FED includes required policies and procedures developed for the transfer process of patients requiring hospital admission. This policy and procedure must be well delineated for the freestanding site. The site must be recognized by CMS as an ED or it is unable (prohibited) to advertise such and cannot bill Medicare for ED visit codes that could be financially challenging depending on the demographics of the location.[6]

Access to Care

As freestanding EDs are often a way for a health system to establish a footprint in an area, many hospitals are combining the site with full-service imaging centers (for ED and outpatient studies) and including small medical office complexes as well.

Although the majority of patients are seen and discharged, between 5% and 10% of patients are transferred for hospital admission or surgical procedures. For FED sites in more rural areas, these facilities can assist emergency medical services (EMS) personnel in stabilizing critically ill patients. Many sites incorporate an onsite helipad to transfer these critical patients.

HOSPITAL SYSTEMS WITH FREESTANDING EMERGENCY DEPARTMENTS

Inova Health System, Fairfax, Va.

Carolinas Healthcare System, Charlotte, N.C.

Hospital Corporation of America (HCA), Virginia, Texas

Swedish Medical Center, Seattle, Wash.

Demographic studies can help determine the best location for FEDs. Areas of rapid population growth, positive housing construction, and per-capita income analysis can assist in the proposition for a FED in a suburban area. These suburban locations help to feed inpatient volume and procedures to the central facility, whereas rural FEDs are often used by healthcare systems to put a new footprint down and provide improved access to care for the population.

The number of FEDs in Texas, specifically in Dallas and Houston, have grown rapidly for both facility-owned and private venture models.[7] Private venture FEDs may or may not participate with insurance or government programs. As with any rapid growth, there will be winners and losers, with some facilities closing the doors due to lack of financial viability.

Care transitions

Similar to urgent care centers, community education is critical for FEDs to be successful—especially with the EMS community. Building trust with the EMS community is important; the site can either become a central part of the region's healthcare system, or it can simply become a temporary stopping point before patients are later shipped to the local hospital. With critical patients, EMS workers may greatly appreciate having an FED that can help stabilize an airway, cardiopulmonary, and/or vascular conditions.

However, it is vital to educate EMS workers on what patients should bypass the site and be directly transported to the main hospital or closest community hospital. These cases often include major trauma, patients obviously requiring admissions, heart attacks, and strokes. As with any hospital-owned site, hospital-owned FEDs have full obligation under Emergency Medical Treatment and Active Labor Act of 1986 (EMTALA) to care for all patients seeking treatment to the capability of that facility. Private venture FEDs may not have this requirement, and they may or may not participate in insurance programs, Medicare, or Medicaid.

One key aspect for hospital-affiliated FEDs is the timely disposition of admitted or critically ill patients. These sites should have considerable priority with acceptance of admissions to the main hospital even over the hospital site ED. The FED has limited capability and cannot provide extended care for admitted patients. Although most transfers are sent to the main hospital, a closer facility may be appropriate depending on the condition and stability of the patient.

It is wise to have some advanced communication with both primary site hospitals and those outside of the healthcare system that may receive patients from the FED. These conversations should take place months in advance and be frequent topics to ensure smooth patient transitions when the time comes. One area that benefits the FED, the patient, and the hospital-based ED is when patients can be directly admitted to a hospitalist service, bypassing the main hospital ED and avoiding clogging ED beds at the main site. Although private ownership FEDs have no obligation under EMTALA (unless Medicare funding is accepted), they will need to have relationships with local hospitals for patients requiring admission. We strongly encourage relationship development similar to that of the hospital-affiliated sites rather than simply calling 911 for a hospital transfer.

Outpatient referrals can also be an obstacle, but FEDs that have an affiliated medical office complex may help ease this challenge. The primary referral areas include primary care (including pediatrics) and orthopedics. Development of an adjacent medical office complex with this in mind helps to feed both programs. Non-hospital-affiliated FEDs should make every effort to develop outpatient referral relations that act to improve transitions of care.

Unique Challenges for the Freestanding Emergency Department

Respiratory therapy

Respiratory therapists typically provide services in hospital EDs, including nebulizer treatments, drawing and running of blood gases, use of CPAP/BiPAP, and management of ventilator patients. Typically, FEDs do not have adequate volume to provide coverage with a reparatory therapist. These skills often fall to the ED staff nurse. We believe that many of these services can be accomplished in the FED, with the most challenging being ventilator management. We would theorize many sites use basic equipment with easy to understand and operate ventilators. The skill of drawing a blood gas may be left to the physician, but certainly the blood gas analyzer should be simple enough for the nurse or laboratory tech to run.

Radiology

The most common needs for radiology include plain films, CT scan, and ultrasound. As discussed previously, hospitals often combine imaging centers with urgent care and FED sites. In addition to providing these types of tests, other capabilities the sites typically offer during business hours include MRI, ultrasound, bone density, and mammography. With the current emergency medicine residency training programs, ED ultrasound may reduce the need for a technologist to be available 24 hours per day, seven days per week. Radiology technicians may also be cross trained in CT without significant difficulty, but this is far more challenging and often not done with ultrasound. Cross training reduces after-hours on-call needs for additional technicians and delays for calling in CT scan personnel. This is obviously more critical for time-sensitive studies including CT scans of the brain for stoke compared to abdominal studies, for example.

Laboratory

It is essential to have a full service lab with the exception of microbiology cultures that can be transferred to the main hospital for incubation and analysis. Although there are many point-of-care tests available, chemistry panels, quantitative drug levels (lanoxin, phenytoin, aspirin, acetaminophen, among others), and basic blood bank testing (type and rh, type and screen) are strongly recommended and require advanced lab instrumentation. In addition, handling blood products is an important topic. For example, you should consider the simple stocking of limited units of O negative for truly emergent situations—especially for those sites in remote locations where patient transfer times are very prolonged.

Pharmacy

Obviously, all of the resuscitation and rapid sequence induction drugs are essential to a FED and may be included in a fully stocked code cart. Rapid sequence induction and sedation agents may include etomidate, ketamine, rocuronium (or vecuronium), succinylcholine, midazolam, and propofol. Nebulizer medication including albuterol and atrovent are also essential for treating both asthma and COPD patients along with methlyprednisolone and dexamethosone. Expanded intravenous or intramuscular antibiotics could include ceftriazone, gentamycin, clindamycin, ampicillin, cefozolin, levofloxacin, and vancomycin. Antiseizure medications should include ativan, valium, phenytoin (or foshenytoin), valproate, and phenobarbital. Octreotide, though rarely used, may be considered for upper gastrointestinal bleeds. Cardiac mediations are often contained in the code cart but should include atropine, adenosine, diltiazem, lidocaine, procainamide, and amiodarone, along with heparin and low molecular weight heparin. As mentioned previously, stocking thrombolytic medications should be considered, but they are costly and may not be needed if patient transfer times are very short. The medications listed above are suggestions and are heavily dependent on local medical practice, medication preferences, and distance to the closet full-service hospital.

Insurance

FED licensing is typically under the same site license as the hospital, which makes Medicare, Medicaid, Blue Cross/Blue Shield, and other insurance participation a less challenging concept. Billing requirements describe Class A and B EDs (defined previously by CMS). Hospital-owned facilities typically see all patients and often operate under the main hospital's license.

It is essential that FED sites undergo state certification in order to ensure that there is a minimum standard of equipment and level of care provided.[8] All sites should be fully integrated components of the healthcare system, including EMS and electronic health records, and have seamless transition of patient care. Provision of minimum standards and integration both help with third-party carrier negotiations for non-hospital-affiliated FEDs. Many Blue Cross/Blue Shield programs reimburse only for professional fees for both urgent care centers and FEDs. Many FEDs have a lower cost structure with fewer bad debts that may reduce overall costs to the patient and insurance carrier.[9] We believe that FEDs should be recognized and fully reimbursed by insurance carriers if they operate at an adequate level and maintain standards similar to hospital-based facilities.

REFERENCES

1.   Huddy, J. 2006. Emergency Department Design: A Practical Guide to Planning for the Future. American College of Physicians, Dallas, Texas.

2.   Katzman, M. 1985. Freestanding Emergency Center: Regulation and Reimbursement. Am J Law Med. 11(1):105–129.

3.   Bush, H. 2008. As Populations Grow, Stand Alone EDs Rise. Hospital and Health Networks. February:20.

4.   Ibid.

5.   Legros, N. 2008. Freestanding Emergency Departments Gain Acceptance by CMS. Reimbursement Advisor. July:3–6.

6. Ibid.

7. Sorele,R. 2011. Breaking News: The Emergence of Freestanding EDs. Emergency Medicine News. 33(6):1, 27.

8. Legros, N. 2008. Freestanding Emergency Departments Gain Acceptance by CMS. Reimbursement Advisor. July:3.

9. Katzman, M. 1985. Freestanding Emergency Center: Regulation and Reimbursement. Am J Law Med. 11(1):105–129.

Retail Clinics

The retail clinic concept evolved in the late 1990s due to the failure of our current healthcare system to provide ready access to efficient low cost-care through emergency departments (ED), and the inability of primary care physicians to provide next-day or same-day appointments or extended office hours. The actual story of retail clinics' origins suggests that a frustrated father was unhappy and unsatisfied with a prolonged wait and high cost of care for his son's strep throat.[1]

Basics of Retail Clinics

The benefit of retail clinics for patients are similar to urgent care centers, including convenient locations, afterhours availability (i.e., nights and weekends), and low prices. The retail clinic model is efficient, low cost, and directed at specific minor illnesses with patient charges starting at about $60 per visit.

The Convenient Care Association (CCA) was developed by retail clinic programs, medical professionals, and others to provide standardization, education, and resources to both the public and its members. Many clinic sites maintain care protocols for the most common diagnoses and conditions. According to the CCA, the top conditions treated in retail clinics in 2008 included sore throat, cold symptoms, flu symptoms, cough, sinus infection, allergies, immunizations, and blood pressure testing.[2]

Locations

The locations of retail clinics are typically in retail pharmacies, grocery stores, and chain stores. The optimum location is in middle to higher income areas in larger retail sites such as supercenter stores. These locations provide enough traffic to sustain the minimum of 15 to 20 patients per day that is needed to maintain economic viability for the clinic site. Site location costs are minimal because most clinics are owned by the retail store and only require one to two rooms. The largest retail chains include RediClinic, MinuteClinic, and Take Care Clinic. These sites promote efficiency (e.g., fast care without appointments), price transparency (e.g., charges are listed on a menu and can be found on the Internet), and lower costs.

Demographics

Studies suggest that this price point targets the insured population with more discretionary income. Some clinics have combated this argument by reducing prices to make it more affordable to the uninsured and underinsured population.[3] Additional demographic information suggests that the majority of the patients seeking retail clinic services do not have an established primary care physician.

Adults often seek care due to this lack of a physician relationship whereas children are brought to retail clinics due to their caregiver's inability to obtain timely appointments for minor illnesses or a physical exam through their pediatrician.

Many clinics discourage repeat visits for continuing care and encourage the medical home model by maintaining physician referral panels for primary care purposes and future visits.[4]

Fenn conducted a study with RediClinic in Houston, which had an association with with Memorial Hermann Healthcare, asking patients where they would go if they had not used the clinic.[5] The findings were not surprising and included the following:

- Emergency department (10%–30%)

- Urgent care center (15%)

- Primary care physician (25%)

- Nowhere (30%)

These results show that clinics are competition for EDs, urgent care centers, and primary care physicians.

Partnerships

Over the past five years, several hospitals and healthcare systems have joined the retail clinic space by partnering with or developing their own retail clinic sites.[6] Health systems can partner with existing clinics by providing consulting services, collaborative practice and practice oversight review (peer review), and allowing bidirectional referral of patients. Health systems can also approach retailers and lease space along with providing the medical provider (i.e., nurse practitioner, physician assistant, and physician), or approach the project as a joint venture.[7]

Legal

Retail clinic legal issues include the existence of the clinic itself. Many states maintain a corporate practice of medicine statute that only allows licensed providers to oversee the care for patients.[8] If the statute stipulates "physician" in its language, retail clinics—owned and operated by the retail store—may have some difficulty even with physician supervision or collaboration. These statutes state that only licensed physicians can be responsible for the oversite or actual care of patients. Obviously, each state has different language and legal counsel with expert opinion should be sought prior to development of a retail clinic program.[9]

For the purposes of this book, we refer to retail clinics as those staffed by nurse practitioners and physician assistants. There is a somewhat different model for the retail clinic as developed by Solantic, a corporate provider of urgent care services. These sites are larger than the retail clinics described previously, maintain a board-certified physician model, but are located in retail areas including airports and malls. They have complete pricing transparency identifying a three-tiered level of service and posting prices for each level along with lists of additional services provided.[10] We consider these in the same category as a full service urgent care model with a wider scope of practice than the nurse practitioner model. These retail clinics have the same philosophy as others including efficiency, price transparency, and competitive prices.

Retail clinics provide a relief valve for the health system by providing access to care for minor ailments. They also, in theory, could become part of an accountable care model by providing patients quick, low-cost, quality care for minor episodic illnesses. Patients can either elect to visit or be referred to these sites by overstretched physician offices, triage call centers (phone), or busy EDs.

Key Takeaway

Clinic owners must abide by state laws regarding healthcare along with medical and nursing boards regarding standards of care. These sites provide efficient service at a lower cost compared to EDs. In addition, retail clinics play a role in disease screening by providing education on hypertension and diabetes along with disease prevention by providing a multitude of immunizations.

REFERENCES

1. Muroff, J. 2009. Retail Healthcare Care: "Taking Stock" of State Responsibilities. J Legal Med. 30:151–179.

2. CCA. Fact Sheet: Physician Oversight retrieved on March 2, 2012, from *http://www.ccaclinics.org.*

3. Muroff, J. 2009. Retail Healthcare Care: "Taking Stock" of State Responsibilities. J Legal Med. 30:151–179.

4. Ibid.

5. Fenn, S. 2008. Integrating CCCs into the Hospital System. Frontiers of Health Service Management. 24(3):33–36.

6. Kaissi, A. 2010. Hospital Affiliated and Hospital-Owned Retail Clinics: Strategic Opportunities and Operational Challenges. J Healthcare Manage. 55(5):324–337.

7. Ibid.

8. Burkle, C. 2011. The Advance of the Retail Health Clinic Market: The Liability Risk Physicians May Potentially Face When Supervising or Collaborating with Other Professionals. Mayo Clinic Proceedings 86(11):1086–1091.

9. Muroff, J. 2009. Retail Healthcare Care: "Taking Stock" of State Responsibilities. J Legal Med. 30:151–179.

10. Bowling, K. 2011. Health Care Goes Retail: Solantic Looks To Retail Marketing Models to Strengthen Its Brand. Spring *www.marketingpower.com*.

15

Urgent Care Centers as Part of Accountable Care Organizations

The United States healthcare system is fragmented for both uninsured and insured patients alike. For example, many Medicare patients seek treatment from multiple specialists often with no primary care physician. There is no "orchestra" leader managing the patient's overall care ensuring that all aspects of their healthcare are being addressed, and that medications are not prescribed which could cause untoward effects or dangerous interactions.

With the passage of the Patient Protection and Affordable Care Act (PPACA) (Section 3022), a significant emphasis has been placed on improving patient care through the development and implementation of best clinical practices, standardization of care, provider accountability for that care, and improved communication. Part of this legislation also includes the formation of accountable care organizations (ACO) that will provide care to at least 5,000 Medicare beneficiaries per defined ACO.

ACO Concept

The ACO concept is not new. In fact, it is similar to the managed care/HMO concept of the 1990s. In that model, an organization was tasked with the responsibility of care for specific populations, and providers were at risk for both costs incurred and outcomes. The difference between the HMO and the ACO is that healthcare providers assume the financial risk versus insurance companies, and there is flexibility with the organizational structure of the ACO.[1]

ACOs will affiliate primary care physicians, specialists, and hospitals working in a network as a physician hospital organization (PHO), independent practice association (IPA), or other similar structure. These networks will be required to communicate through a common electronic health record (EHR). The development of "certified" EHRs has also been encouraged by the Centers for Medicare & Medicaid Services (CMS) through its meaningful use regulations that strive to improve healthcare quality, safety, and efficiency through the promotion of health information technology.

THREE PART AIM OF ACOS[2]

- Improved individual care

- Better health for the population (focus on wellness reducing the cost of disease)

- Lower costs (reduce duplicate testing, reduce unnecessary referral to specialty care, avoid unnecessary admissions)

Up to 15% of the Medicare population is admitted to hospitals each year. Some healthcare experts suggest that more aggressive outpatient care strategies can reduce this number. In addition, improved coordination post hospital discharge may prevent the 20% readmission rate for the Medicare population. ACO goals include reducing unnecessary hospitalization, eliminating duplicate testing, and preventing avoidable complications.[3] The ACO concept incorporates the medical home model with primary care physicians, and the concept has greater focus on outcomes and avoiding preventable costs. Savings to Medicare from reduction in costs, preventing avoidable complications, duplicate testing, etc., are then shared back with the ACO group and its providers.

ACO Structure

The ACO structure becomes the "parent" organization over providers (i.e., primary care and specialists), hospitals, and home healthcare agencies. Like any good parent, the ACO develops the rules with clinical guidelines; pharmacy and therapeutic committee reviews to develop best practice patterns of medication use, evidence-based guidelines, group purchasing programs for approving/bulk purchasing of medical devices and supplies; and enforces compliance with inclusion or exclusion of providers, vendors, and facilities.

The main goal of the PPACA is to improve care, but it also strives for financial accountability that is overseen by CMS and the U.S. Department of Health and Human Services with an expected savings of $960 million dollars in the first three years. This corresponds to less than 1% of the Medicare budget.[4]

ACO GOALS
1. Focus on patients/link payment to outcomes
2. Improve safety/quality
3. Make healthcare more affordable
4. Avoid duplication of services
5. Focus on best practices/evidence-based medicine
FINANCIAL BENEFITS FOR ACOS
1. Cost saving in test avoidance (better margins with fewer tests)
2. Shared financial benefit from Medicare "savings"
3. Improved market position for high performers (more business)
4. Improved patient satisfaction resulting in more business
CHRONIC HEALTH CONDITIONS BEING TARGETED
1. Hypertension
2. Diabetes
3. Asthma/COPD
4. Kidney disease
5. Congestive heart failure
6. Coronary artery disease

The Healthcare Executive's Guide to Urgent Care Centers and Freestanding EDs

Networks of primary care providers, specialists, and hospitals share the financial responsibility for delivering quality care to a minimum of 5,000 Medicare beneficiaries by coordinating and allocating resources for care. The ACO would be paid bonuses for meeting quality benchmarks (performance with acute myocardial infarction, pneumonia, diabetes, hypertension control, etc.) and controlling costs of care. There is continued—and increased focus—on prevention and management of chronic disease. If ACOs don't meet the expected standard, they will not be awarded any savings and could be eliminated from the program.

Because Medicare Part D covers most medications for the elderly, the new program will place a large focus on drug utilization by providers (evidence-based medicine) and patient medication compliance. As a result, hospital formularies will likely be reduced focusing on fewer agents choosing and negotiating with suppliers for the lowest system price.

Obviously, the costs for developing ACO infrastructure will be quite sizable. Savings and bonuses may not cover the costs of the infrastructure, implementation, and ongoing management of data. Similar to HMOs of the 90s, providers may be "rewarded" for keeping patients healthier and out of the hospital. The program may improve coordination of care by requiring all providers in the ACO to utilize a common EHR.

Documentation and Electronic Health Records

Documentation is key to communication and has been a major challenge for the healthcare system as a whole. Records between providers, hospitals, and other healthcare facilities are often not accessible, mergable, or electronically transferable (with any significant ease). The concept of "meaningful use" was developed by CMS and basically translates to a certified health record meeting specific objectives. Some of the requirements for EHRs include electronic prescribing, electronic physician order entry, and electronic health information

---

BASIC CONCEPTS FOR AN ACO[5]

1. Formal legal structure to receive and distribute shared savings

2. Sufficient primary care providers to care for 5,000 (minimum) assigned beneficiaries

3. Three-year participation

4. Maintain adequate information on providers

5. Leadership and management structure including clinical and administrative systems

6. Process definitions

   a. Evidence-based medicine

   b. Report quality and cost data (prescribing, PQRI results)

7. Demonstrate that ACO provides patient-centered care

Results include:

1. Reduce supplier access to providers (more time with patients), greater bulk purchasing and consolidation of practices

2. Manufacturers may present to P&T committees to demonstrate value and purchase decisions made at that level (rather than by the specific provider)

3. Formal treatment protocols and guidelines, physician will have less autonomy

4. Clinical outcomes and cost data for all

---

including current allergies, medications, problem lists, and results of diagnostic tests. CMS offers incentives for installing EHRs to healthcare systems, hospitals, and individual providers. The intent is to improve the availability of health record, reduce errors, and improve communication between providers.

Specific physician and MLP incentives are available either through Medicare or Medicaid participation, but not both programs. Payments under Medicare are a maximum of $44,000 over five years and with Medicaid a maximum of $63,750 over six years.[6] In order to participate under the Medicaid program, the physician practice must care for at least 30% Medicaid patients. By the year 2015, those providers not demonstrating meaningful use may have reimbursement reduced to a maximum of 5%.

Each provider must attest to 15 core measures and utilize five of 10 menu sets. Some of these core measures include drug–drug interaction checks, active medication list, patient allergies, documentation of vital signs, and smoking history. The menu sets including incorporating a lab results area for each chart, sending patient reminders for follow-up care, providing summaries of care during transitions to other providers, and implementation of drug formulary checks. Further information can be obtained from *www.cms.gov/Regulations-and-guidance/ Legislation/EHRIncentivePrograms*.

Urgent Centers and ACOs

Urgent care centers provide a critical relief valve for primary care offices and overcrowded EDs and could be an integral part of any ACO. With cost-effective care, use of EHRs, and affiliation with hospitals and healthcare systems, urgent care centers become a competitive force augmenting the function of the ACO. They need to continue to focus on episodic injury and illness care.

Hospital-based and affiliated sites can provide the transition back to the community by providing postdischarge follow-ups for hospitalized patients ensuring that they understand the care plan, have filled and are taking prescriptions correctly, and have a medical home to be referred to (or the center can set up the next appointment with a medical home). In addition, they can offer services for wound checks, antibiotic dosages for cellulitis, follow-up appointments from patients seen in the ED, and provide "warfarin" clinic services, among others.

Key Takeaway

ACOs require seamless transition in patient care, communication via an EHR, and demonstrated outcome improvement for patient participants. In order to accomplish this task, we need to start merging healthcare "silos" to become successful in the future. Urgent care centers can be an integral component of these programs by providing additional access specifically for minor illness and injury that reduces the burden to the organizations' physician practices and emergency departments. In addition, this can be accomplished at a cost-effective price.

REFERENCES

1. Berger, E. Emergency Physicians Face Uncertainty in Accountable Care Organizations. Annals of Emergency Medicine 57(4):13A.

2. Berwick, D. Launching Accountable Care Organizations-The Proposed Rule for Medicare Shared Savings Program. N Engl J Med. 364(16):e32.

3. Kocker, R., Sahni, N. 2010. Physicians versus Hospitals as Leaders of Accountable Care Organizations. N Engl J Med. 263(27):2579–2582.

4. Gold, J. 2011. Accountable Care Organizations, Explained. Retrieved May 3, 2011, from *www.npr.org*.

5. Kocker, R., Sahni, N. 2010. Physicians versus Hospitals as Leaders of Accountable Care Organizations. N Engl J Med. 263(27):2579–2582.

6. McDonald, E. 2011. Planning for Meaningful Use? The Clock is Ticking. J Urgent Care Med. September:21–24.

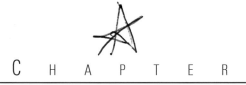

The Ideal Urgent Care Clinic

Similar to the ABCs in emergency medicine, the ideal urgent care clinic starts with the fundamental building blocks of a financial plan and data acquisition. This is followed by determining location opportunities and financing. The facility staff is then recruited along with arranging an equipment list and any site renovation considerations. As the opening approaches and the provider team is selected, managed care negotiations begin for contracting and enrollment. Finally, the doors open and the adventure begins.

Planning the "I Have a Dream" Clinic

The first step to building our version of an ideal clinic is to develop a solid financial plan and proforma, which enables you to obtain the necessary capital and line of credit. Securing financing and credit enables you to open the doors and funds payroll for the first year.

In our organizations, we provide the physician/midlevel staffing only with the major capital requirements provided by the healthcare system. With independent clinic start ups, the minimum capital required ranges from $500,000–$750,000;

this includes finances for site renovation, equipment, and other costs. In addition, lines of credit through banks (or other avenues) are required to fund payroll and operating costs for the first six months up to one year. This is less of an issue with hospital-affiliated facilities in that facility participation with insurance products reduces accounts receivable and billing delays.

Location

The site selection should occur six to nine months prior to opening day, depending on construction needs. The target opening date would ideally be June or July to provide adequate time to prepare for the peak flu season, which most often occurs from January through March. Then you should select a high-traffic location (characterized by more than 25,000 vehicles passing on the facing street front per day). The clinic should also be near retail shopping and surrounded by home owners with annual incomes greater than $50,000. The site size of 3,500 square feet includes five treatment rooms, two procedure rooms, a digital radiography (DR) x-ray system with PACS, an integrated electronic medical record (EMR), and a waive testing lab.

Target market

The patient population includes minor illnesses and injuries, sports and school physicals, and possibly some travel medicine, including immunizations. An occupational medicine practice with drug screening (e.g., Department of Transportation and Federal Aviation Administration physicals, audiometry, PFT, and FIT testing) evaluates initial injuries and provides follow-up care for patients until they are released back to work. We would provide Healthcare Insurance Portability and Accountability Act of 1996–compliant communication within 24 hours of the patient's visit to each patient's primary care provider.

Having a minor illness and injury focus provides for the majority of the clinic's business. We, however, maintain basic and initial advanced life support capability with staff training and certification, a functional cardiac monitor/defibrillator/ pacer, airway/ventilation equipment, and necessary basic resuscitation drugs. In addition, we would have a close relationship with local EMS and the emergency department (ED) to create seamless transition of patient care.

Recruitment

The recruiting processes should start at least 90 days before preopening. The center's mission and core values statement should be used during the recruiting process, and these values should be delineated to all staff to develop a team harmony. Key aspects of the site's missions, values, and goals would be reinforced monthly and during all clinic meetings.

Managed care

Managed care negotiations and developing strong relations with the provider enrollment departments begins with provider paperwork flowing just before opening to expedite participation. Securing Medicare participation should occur as soon as provider numbers are obtained. Initially, the clinic may start accepting cash collections only and charging amounts equal to copays until insurance plan participation is finalized. We would recruit an experienced office or practice manager to help with this process along with contracting an experienced billing company.

Certification

The center should apply for certification through the Urgent Care Association of America (UCAOA), which requires facilities to meet specific standards. UCAOA also offers a pre-opening certification designation. Centers should also consider accreditation by The Joint Commission that attests to meeting certain standards and other medical performance goals.

Marketing

Hospital affiliation or cobranding often increases patient traffic but is not required and occurs in less than about 35% of facilities. Marketing should occur, for the most part, by word of mouth. But the site's medical director should visit all local primary and pediatric practice offices to market for afterhours care, meet with the local ED director to market for overflow and postvisit referrals, and meet with local sporting teams for physical examination and potential sponsorship of youth leagues. In addition, the center would have a large sign visible from the road and lit at night along with an LCD providing community information, center "specials," and other information. Further, it should do a directed ZIP code mailing for a 10-mile radius, marketing the center and educating potential patients regarding the services and care abilities of the site.

Clinic management

The site would employ (or contract with) a designated physician medical director for oversight of the physicians, nurse practitioners, and physicians assistants. The site would be overseen by an experienced nurse with additional management skills. His or her responsibilities include recruiting/hiring staff (i.e., technicians, nurses, and clerical staff), ordering and tracking supplies, assessing medical quality, managing compliance, and doing some marketing. This position would ensure the clinic runs successfully.

As an integral part of the team, registration staff should verify all insurance information and addresses, obtain preauthorization if needed, and collect all copays and deductibles. It is vital to remember that more employers are moving to higher deductible plans, so the center may need to collect the entire cost of the visit at the time of service for many of these health plans. This also applies to those patients with medical savings accounts. Failure to collect payment at the time of service makes it very difficult to collect later. The facility should have a credit and debit card machine for payment at time of service.

The registration staff should be well paid and have goals and financial incentives as an integral part of their job. In addition, close attention should be paid to reconciling cash collected for these services. Larger sums of cash should be quickly placed in a "drop" safe and taken to the bank for deposit on a daily basis.

Facility design

The facility should be cosmetically appealing but doesn't need design extremes to conserve capital. Patients should be taken immediately to the treatment area when a bed is available. Provider staffing should target volumes not exceeding three patients per hour per provider. Higher staffing ratios result in delays in delivering care to patients, clinical errors, and poor satisfaction (unless all of the patients are very low acuity). The average visit duration for patients to be seen and discharged should be less than 75 minutes. All patients should be contacted the next day to assess the patient's clinical condition and determine satisfaction.

The clinic should position itself as an integral part of the healthcare system and accountable care organizations. Care provided should be efficient, cost-effective, and integrated with the local healthcare system. Quality patient care and customer service excellence should exist as the primary core value of the site.

Example Equipment Cost List

	NUMBER	ITEM COSTS	COSTS
Waiting room			
Chairs	20	$150	$3,000
End table	3	$250	$750
Plasma screen TV	1	$1,000	$1,000
Trash can	2	$50	$100
Water dispenser	1	$200	$200
Health information table	1	$350	$350
Artwork	3	$600	$1,800
Information board	1	$200	$200
Total			$7,400

	NUMBER	ITEM COSTS	COSTS
Registration			
Credit/debit card reader	1	$250	$250
Computer	2	$1,200	$2,400
Chairs (staff)	2	$500	$1,000
Chair (patient)	2	$250	$500
Money drop safe	1	$250	$250
Phone	2	$400	$800
Printer	2	$200	$400
Copier	1	$5,000	$5,000
Label printer			0
Total			$10,600

The Healthcare Executive's Guide to Urgent Care Centers and Freestanding EDs 215

Appendix A

	NUMBER	INDIVIDUAL ITEM COSTS	TOTAL COSTS
Triage			
Triple glove holder	1	$65	$65
Trash can	1	$65	$65
Desk	1	$200	$200
Patient chair	1	$150	$150
Provider stool	1	$200	$200
Oto/ophthalmoscope	1	$600	$600
Computer	1	$1,200	$1,200
Vital signs machine	1		0
Thermometer	1		0
Adult scale	1		0
Infant scale	1		0
Phone	1	$200	$200
Digital clock	1	$45	$45
Artwork	1	$200	$200
Total			$2,925

Exam room			
Triple glove holder	7	$65	$455
Trash can	7	$25	$175
Exam table	7	$1,000	$7,000
Visitor chair	14	$150	$2,100
Provider stool	7	$200	$1,400
Oto/ophthalmoscope	7	$600	$4,200
Computer	1	$1,200	$1,200
Plasma television	1	$500	$500
Digital clock	7	$45	$315
Foot stools	7	$50	$350
Mayo stands	7	$450	$3,150
Artwork	7	$250	$1,750
Total			$22,595

	NUMBER	INDIVIDUAL ITEM COSTS	TOTAL COSTS
Procedure room			
Portable procedure light	1	$1,000	$1,000
Triple glove holder	1	$65	$65
Trash can	1	$25	$25
Procedure gurney	1	$5,000	$5,000
Visitor chair	2	$150	$300
Provider stool	2	$200	$400
Oto/ophthalmoscope	1	$600	$600
Computer	1	$1,200	$1,200
Plasma television	1	$500	$500
Artwork	2	$250	$500
Total			$9,590

	NUMBER	INDIVIDUAL ITEM COSTS	TOTAL COSTS
Nurse/provider station			
Computer	3	$1,200	$3,600
Phones	3	$400	$1,200
Shred bin	1	$50	$50
Chairs	3	$200	$600
Printer	3	$250	$750
Fax machine	1	$300	$300
Digital clock	1	$45	$45
PACS reading station	1	$10,000	$10,000
Total			$16,545

Appendix A

	NUMBER	INDIVIDUAL ITEM COSTS	TOTAL COSTS
Utility/storage			
Trash can	1	$100	$100
Biohazard trash can	1	$100	$100
Mop/bucket	1	$50	$50
Optional equipment			
AED/defib	1	$1,750	$1,750
IV pumps	3	$1,600	$4,800
EKG machine	1	$13,250	$13,250
Portable suction machine	1	$500	$500
Wheelchair	1	$500	$500
Wheelchair/bariatric	1	$1,000	$1,000
Security camera/system			
Total			$21,800
Office			
Desk	1	$400	$400
Chair	1	$250	$250
Phone	1	$400	$400
File cabinet	1	$300	$300
Computer	1	$1,200	$1,200
Printer	1	$500	$500
Bookcase	1	$400	$400
Bulletin boards	2	$75	$150
Trash can	1	$50	$50
Artwork	1	$250	$3,650
Lab station (draw only)			
Chair, bariatric phleb	1	$1,046	$1,046
Supply stand	1	$559	$559
Computer	1	$1,900	$1,900
Bar code printer	1	$750	$750

The Healthcare Executive's Guide to Urgent Care Centers and Freestanding EDs

	NUMBER	INDIVIDUAL ITEM COSTS	TOTAL COSTS
Bar code scanner	1	$200	$200
Telephone	1	$400	$400
Chair, office, vinyl	1	$200	$200
Tube rack	1	$200	$200
Total			$5,255

Centrifuge	1	$3,794	$3,794
Refrigerator	1		$0
Freezer, small cube	1		$0
Computer	1	$1,200	$1,200
Bar code printer	1	$750	$750
Bar code scanner	1	$200	$200
Telephone	1	$400	$400
Printer/copier/fax	1	$350	$350
Chair, office, vinyl	1	$200	$200
Istat	1	$9,500	$9,500
Urine dipstick reader	1	$1,800	$1,800
Total			$18,194

Break room			
Table	1	$450	$450
Chairs	8	$150	$1,200
Bulletin boards	2	$100	$200
Refrigerator	1	$450	$450
Microwave	1	$200	$200
Toaster	1	$90	$90
Bookcase	1	$500	$500
Trash can	2	$50	$100
HR bulletin board	1	$400	$400
Phone	1	$400	$400
Coffee pot	1	$198	$198
TV/DVD	1	$500	$500
Total			$4,688

Example Supply Inventory List

Items Table List Report

dbtrec

Limits: Omni Site+ID equals OHURGENT

Omni Site+ID	Item ID #	Item Description	Control Level	Par Level Qty	Qty On Hand	Stock Type
OHURGENT	BLOO-214	ACCU-CHEK (50'S) 1EA BOTL	6	2	1	U
OHURGENT	ACET-16	ACETAMIN/CODEINE 300/30MG 1EA TAB	3	20	15	U
OHURGENT	ACET15EL	ACETAMIN/CODEINE UD LIQUID 15ML ELX	3	5	5	U
OHURGENT	ACET120S14	ACETAMINOPHEN 120MG SUPP	6	10	11	U
OHURGENT	ACET650S	ACETAMINOPHEN 160MG/5ML 20.3ML UDC	6	10	10	U
OHURGENT	ACET325S13	ACETAMINOPHEN 325MG SUPP	6	10	10	U
OHURGENT	ACET-928	ACETAMINOPHEN 325MG TAB	6	25	46	U
OHURGENT	ACET650S14	ACETAMINOPHEN 650MG SUPP	6	10	9	U
OHURGENT	ACET100D6	ACETAMINOPHEN 80MG/0.8ML 15ML DROPS	6	5	4	U
OHURGENT	ACET500T62	ACETAMINOPHEN ES 500MG TAB	6	25	36	U
OHURGENT	ACTI50OR2	ACTIDOSE-AQ 50G/240ML 240ML LIQ	6	2	2	U
OHURGENT	ACYC200C4	ACYCLOVIR 200MG CAP	6	10	10	U
OHURGENT	ADEN3VIA4	ADENOSINE 3MG/1ML 2ML INJ	6	0	4	U
OHURGENT	ALBU2.5V13	ALBUTEROL 0.083% UD 2.5MG/3ML 3ML NEB	0	10	16	U
OHURGENT	ALBU8HFA2	ALBUTEROL HFA 90 MCG 8G INH	0	10	7	U
OHURGENT	IPRA3AMP13	ALBUTEROL&IPRATROPIUM 3ML NEB	0	15	8	U
OHURGENT	ALPRO.2555	ALPRAZolam 0.25MG TAB	4	10	8	U
OHURGENT	AMLO5TAB93	amLODIPine 5MG TAB	6	10	10	U
OHURGENT	AMMO1AMP4	AMMONIA AMPULE 0.33ML INH	6	10	6	S
OHURGENT	AMOX-242	AMOX/CLAVULANATE 500MG TAB	6	10	8	U
OHURGENT	AMOX-326	AMOX/CLAVULANATE 875MG TAB	6	10	6	U
OHURGENT	AMOX250C4	AMOXICILLIN 250MG CAP	6	10	8	U
OHURGENT	AMOX250S16	AMOXICILLIN 250MG/5ML 80ML SUS	6	300	300	U
OHURGENT	AMOX125S4	AMOXICILLIN 25MG/1ML 80ML SUS	6	320	320	U
OHURGENT	AMOX-234	AMOXICILLIN 500MG CAP	6	10	8	U
OHURGENT	AMOX200S15	AMOXICILLIN/CLAV 200MG/5ML 50ML SUSP	6	200	200	U
OHURGENT	AMOX400S66	AMOXICILLIN/CLAV 400MG/5ML 50ML SUSP	6	150	88	U
OHURGENT	AMPI3VIA3	AMPICILLIN/SULBACTAM ADD-VAN 3G INJ	6	2	2	U
OHURGENT	ANTI10DR2	ANTIPY/BENZOCAINE OTIC 10ML SOL	6	5	4	U
OHURGENT	HYPR15DR5	ARTIFICIAL TEARS 15ML SOL	6	5	3	U
OHURGENT	ASPI-674	ASPIRIN BABY CHEW 81MG TAB	6	36	72	U
OHURGENT	ASPI-627	ASPIRIN EC 81MG TAB	6	20	20	U
OHURGENT	ATRO0.1D3	ATROPINE SULF 1MG/10ML 10ML SYRINGE	6	0	4	S
OHURGENT	AZIT200S5	AZITHROMYCIN 200MG/5ML 30ML SUSP	6	150	122	U
OHURGENT	AZIT250T81	AZITHROMYCIN 250MG TAB	6	15	12	U
OHURGENT	NEOM1PAC2	BAC/NEO/POLY 0.9G PKT	6	0	0	U
OHURGENT	PIPE180S	BEDDING SPRAY 142G AER	6	2	2	U
OHURGENT	PHEN-255	BELLA ALK/PB 16.2MG/5ML 10ML SYRINGE	6	3	3	U
OHURGENT	TETR56SP	BENZOCAINE(Cetacaine) 14% ORAL 56G AER	6	2	3	U
OHURGENT	BENZ100C43	BENZONATATE 100MG CAP	6	10	9	U
OHURGENT	BISA10SU21	BISACODYL 10MG SUPP	6	10	10	U
OHURGENT	BISA5TAB40	BISACODYL 5MG TAB	6	10	9	U
OHURGENT	BUDE0.253	BUDESONIDE NEB 0.25MG/2ML 2ML SUS	0	10	10	U

11/21/2011   15:11:44   **Items Table List Report**   Page 2

Limits: Omni Site+ID equals OHURGENT

Omni Site+ID	Item ID #	Item Description	Control Level	Par Level Qty	Qty On Hand	Stock Type
OHURGENT	BUDE0.5A2	BUDESONIDE NEB 0.5MG/2ML 2ML SUS	0	10	10	U
OHURGENT	BUPI2.5V8	BUPIVACAINE 0.25% 50ML INJ	6	10	10	U
OHURGENT	CARB15DR13	CARBAMIDE PEROX EAR DROPS 15ML OTIC	6	5	5	U
OHURGENT	CEFA1VIA9	ceFAZolin 1000MG INJ	6	5	4	U
OHURGENT	CEFA1VIA5	ceFAZolin ADD-VAN 1G INJ	6	5	4	U
OHURGENT	CEFD125S6	CEFDINIR 125MG/5ML 60ML SUS	6	120	119	U
OHURGENT	CEFD300C4	CEFDINIR 300MG CAP	6	10	13	U
OHURGENT	CEFT1VIA24	cefTRIAXone 1000MG INJ	6	5	4	U
OHURGENT	CEFT500V13	cefTRIAXone 500MG INJ	6	5	4	U
OHURGENT	CEFT1VIA16	cefTRIAXone ADD-VAN 1G INJ	6	4	3	U
OHURGENT	CEFU250T53	CEFUROXIME 250MG TAB	6	10	10	U
OHURGENT	CEPH250C	CEPHALEXIN 250MG CAP	6	10	10	U
OHURGENT	CHLO118L3	CHLORHEXIDINE 4OZ LIQ	6	5	5	U
OHURGENT	CIPR10DR	CIPRO HC OTIC 10ML 1EA SUSP	6	2	2	U
OHURGENT	CIPR250T6	CIPROFLOXACIN 250MG TAB	6	10	9	U
OHURGENT	CIPR500T6	CIPROFLOXACIN 500MG TAB	6	10	10	U
OHURGENT	CLAR250S11	CLARITHROMYCIN 250MG/5ML 50ML SUS	6	100	100	U
OHURGENT	CLAR-12	CLARITHROMYCIN 500MG TAB	6	10	8	U
OHURGENT	CLIN150C17	CLINDAMYCIN 150MG CAP	6	10	8	U
OHURGENT	CLIN150V11	CLINDAMYCIN 600MG/4ML 4ML VIAL	6	10	7	U
OHURGENT	CLON0.1T42	cloNIDine 0.1MG TAB	6	10	8	U
OHURGENT	COLC0.6T3	COLCHICINE 0.6MG TAB	6	6	6	U
OHURGENT	CYCL-18	CYCLOBENZAPRINE 10MG TAB	6	10	9	U
OHURGENT	DEXT100037	D5 /0.45%NS 1000ML INJ	6	4	4	U
OHURGENT	METH40VI18	DEPO-MEDROL 40MG/1ML 1ML INJ	6	8	15	U
OHURGENT	DEXA1TAB2	DEXAMETHASONE 1MG TAB	6	6	6	U
OHURGENT	DEXA4VIA12	DEXAMETHASONE INJ 4MG/1ML 1ML INJ	6	5	5	U
OHURGENT	DEXA4VIA2	DEXAMETHASONE INJ 4MG/1ML 5ML INJ	6	5	3	U
OHURGENT	D5WILVIS	DEXTROSE 5%/WATER 1000ML IV	6	4	4	U
OHURGENT	D5500VIS	DEXTROSE 5%/WATER 500ML INJ	6	2	2	U
OHURGENT	DEXT50DI4	DEXTROSE 50% ABBJ 50ML INJ	6	0	3	U
OHURGENT	DIAZ5DIS4	DIAZEPAM 10MG/2ML 2ML INJ	4	10	9	U
OHURGENT	DIAZ-150	DIAZEPAM 5MG TAB	4	10	8	U
OHURGENT	DIGO125T60	DIGOXIN 125MCG TAB	6	5	5	U
OHURGENT	DIPH12.511	DIPHENHIST 25MG/10ML 10ML UDC	6	10	7	U
OHURGENT	DIPH-113	diphenhydrAMINE 25MG TAB	6	10	6	U
OHURGENT	DIPH50VI3	diphenhydrAMINE 50MG/1ML 1ML INJ	6	6	4	S
OHURGENT	DIPH1TAB91	DIPHENOXYLATE/ATROPINE 2.5MG TAB	5	10	10	U
OHURGENT	DOCU50LI	DOCUSATE SODIUM 100MG/10ML 10ML UDC	6	8	8	U
OHURGENT	DOXY100C53	DOXYCYCLINE 100MG CAP	6	10	10	U
OHURGENT	DOXY100V	DOXYCYCLINE 100MG INJ	6	4	4	U
OHURGENT	ENOX100D	ENOXAPARIN 100MG/1ML 1ML INJ	6	2	2	U
OHURGENT	ENOX40DI	ENOXAPARIN 40MG/0.4ML 0.4ML INJ	6	3	3	U
OHURGENT	ENOX80DI	ENOXAPARIN 80MG/0.8ML 0.8ML INJ	6	3	3	U
OHURGENT	EPIN0.1D4	EPINEPHrine 1MG/10ML 10ML SYRINGE	6	6	10	S
OHURGENT	EPIN0.3P2	EPINEPHrine PEN 0.3MG INJ	6	2	2	U

Appendix B

Limits: Omni Site+ID equals OHURGENT

Omni Site+ID	Item ID #	Item Description	Control Level	Par Level Qty	Qty On Hand	Stock Type
OHURGENT	EPIN0.153	EPINEPHrine PEN JR 0.15MG INJ	6	2	2	U
OHURGENT	ERYT500T2	ERYTHROMYCIN 500MG TAB	6	6	6	U
OHURGENT	BUTA1TAB9	ESGIC 50/325/40MG 1EA TAB	6	10	20	U
OHURGENT	SOD120IR2	EYE IRRIGATION 118ML SOL	6	6	5	U
OHURGENT	FAMO10TA9	FAMOTIDINE 10MG TAB	6	10	10	U
OHURGENT	FLUC100T5	FLUCONAZOLE 100MG TAB	6	10	10	U
OHURGENT	FLUT16SP	FLUTICASONE NASAL 50MCG 16G SPRAY	6	3	3	U
OHURGENT	FURO40TA8	FUROSEMIDE 40MG TAB	6	10	10	U
OHURGENT	FURO10DI9	FUROSEMIDE SYR 40MG/4ML 4ML INJ	6	5	5	U
OHURGENT	GENT3.5O4	GENTAMICIN 0.3% OPHTH 3.5G OINT	6	4	2	U
OHURGENT	GENT5DRO7	GENTAMICIN 0.3% OPHTH 5ML SOLN	6	4	4	U
OHURGENT	GLUC1VIA	GLUCAGON 1MG KIT	6	2	2	S
OHURGENT	GLYC1SUP14	GLYCERIN ADULT 1EA SUPP	6	5	7	U
OHURGENT	GLYC1SUP20	GLYCERIN INFANT 1SUPP SUPP	6	5	10	U
OHURGENT	GUAI100L14	guaiFENesin 100MG/5ML 10ML UDC	6	10	10	U
OHURGENT	GUAI10LI	guaiFENesin AC 10ML SYRUP	5	8	6	U
OHURGENT	GUAI10SY	guaiFENesin DM 10ML UDC	6	5	5	U
OHURGENT	GUAI600T13	guaiFENesin LA 600MG TAB	6	6	6	U
OHURGENT	HYDR-2054	HYDROCHLOROTHIAZIDE 25MG TAB	6	10	6	U
OHURGENT	HYDR1TAB71	HYDROcodone/ACETAMIN 5/500M 1TAB TAB	3	25	23	U
OHURGENT	HYDR30CR9	HYDROCORTISONE CREAM 1% 30G CRE	6	4	3	U
OHURGENT	HYDR474S	HYDROGEN PEROXIDE 473ML SOL	6	5	5	U
OHURGENT	HYDR473S5	HYDROMET SYRUP 5/1.5MG 5ML SYRINGE	4	8	8	U
OHURGENT	HYDR25CA26	hydrOXYzine 25MG TAB	6	10	8	U
OHURGENT	HYDR25VI	hydrOXYzine 25MG/1ML 1ML INJ	6	6	5	U
OHURGENT	IBUP-55	IBUPROFEN 200MG TAB	6	15	21	U
OHURGENT	IBUP200SUS	IBUPROFEN 200MG/10ML 10ML UDC	6	10	7	U
OHURGENT	IBUP-1147	IBUPROFEN 400MG TAB	6	20	14	U
OHURGENT	IBUP600T4	IBUPROFEN 600MG TAB	6	10	10	U
OHURGENT	NOVOLINR	INS REGULAR U-100 100UNIT/1ML 10ML INJ	6	2000	2000	U
OHURGENT	DEXT37.52	INSTA GLUCOSE 37.5G GEL	6	5	5	S
OHURGENT	IPRA0.2S12	IPRATROPIUM 0.5MG/2.5ML 2.5ML NEB SOL	0	10	22	U
OHURGENT	KETO30VI	KETOROLAC 30MG/1ML 1ML INJ	6	10	10	U
OHURGENT	KETO60VI5	KETOROLAC 60MG/2ML 2ML INJ	6	10	12	U
OHURGENT	LABE5VIA	LABETALOL 5MG/1ML 20ML INJ	6	3	3	U
OHURGENT	RING100013	LACTATED RINGERS 1000ML INJ	6	6	6	U
OHURGENT	LETGEL	LET GEL 1ML SYRINGE	6	10	9	U
OHURGENT	LEVA0.634	LEVALBUTEROL 0.63MG/3ML 3ML NEB	0	24	16	U
OHURGENT	LEVA1.256	LEVALBUTEROL 1.25MG/3ML 3ML NEB	0	24	24	U
OHURGENT	LEVO250T12	LEVOFLOXACIN 250MG TAB	6	10	6	U
OHURGENT	LEVO500T26	LEVOFLOXACIN 500MG TAB	6	10	7	U
OHURGENT	LIDO10VI15	LIDOCAINE 1% INJ 20ML MDV	6	10	18	U
OHURGENT	LIDO100D2	LIDOCAINE 100MG/5ML 5ML SYRINGE	6	4	4	S
OHURGENT	LIDO30JE4	LIDOCAINE 2% 30G JELLY	6	2	2	U
OHURGENT	LIDO20VI16	LIDOCAINE 2% INJ 20ML MDV	6	10	0	U
OHURGENT	LIDO20SO	LIDOCAINE 2% VISC 20MG/1ML 100ML SOL	6	0	8	U

The Healthcare Executive's Guide to Urgent Care Centers and Freestanding EDs

11/21/2011 15:11:44 **Items Table List Report**   Page 4

Limits: Omni Site+ID equals OHURGENT

Omni Site+ID	Item ID #	Item Description	Control Level	Par Level Qty	Qty On Hand	Stock Type
OHURGENT	LIDO20SO2	LIDOCAINE 2% VISCOUS 20ML UDC	6	8	7	U
OHURGENT	LIDO30VI6	LIDOCAINE/EPI 2% 1:100000 30ML INJ	6	4	2	U
OHURGENT	LISI10TA9	LISINOPRIL 10MG TAB	6	10	8	U
OHURGENT	LOPE2CAP44	LOPERAMIDE 2MG CAP	6	10	10	U
OHURGENT	LORA1TAB74	LORazepam 1MG TAB	4	10	5	U
OHURGENT	LORA2DIS5	LORazepam 2MG/1ML 1ML INJ	4	2	4	U
OHURGENT	MAGN30OR	MAALOX/MYLANTA SUB 30ML UDC	6	10	8	U
OHURGENT	MECL25TA95	MECLIZINE 25MG TAB	6	10	6	U
OHURGENT	MEPE50DI	MEPERIDINE 50MG/1ML 1ML INJ	2	10	11	U
OHURGENT	METF500T55	metFORMIN 500MG TAB	6	0	0	U
OHURGENT	METH125V13	methylPREDNISolone 125MG INJ	6	10	9	U
OHURGENT	METH40VI13	methylPREDNISolone 40MG INJ	6	10	9	U
OHURGENT	METO-76	METOCLOPRAMIDE 10MG TAB	6	10	10	U
OHURGENT	METO5VIA10	METOCLOPRAMIDE 5MG/1ML 2ML INJ	6	10	7	U
OHURGENT	METO25TA23	METOPROLOL 25MG TAB	6	10	10	U
OHURGENT	METR-52	metroNIDAZOLE 500MG TAB	6	10	6	U
OHURGENT	MIDA2SYR	MIDAZOLAM ORAL 2MG/1ML 1ML SYRUP	4	5	5	U
OHURGENT	MAGN40OO7	MILK OF MAGNESIA 30ML UDC	6	5	5	U
OHURGENT	MINE480O10	MINERAL OIL 480ML OIL	6	2	2	U
OHURGENT	MORP10DI	MORPHINE SULF 10MG/1ML 1ML INJ	2	10	15	U
OHURGENT	MORP2DIS	MORPHINE SULF 2MG/1ML 1ML INJ	2	10	6	U
OHURGENT	NALB10AM	NALBUPHINE 10MG/1ML 1ML INJ	6	10	8	U
OHURGENT	NAPR500T50	NAPROXEN 500MG TAB	6	10	9	U
OHURGENT	NEOM3.5O2	NEO/POLY/BAC/HC OPHTH 3.5G OINT	6	4	3	U
OHURGENT	NEO/5DRO7	NEO/POLY/DEX 0.1% OPHTH 5ML SUS	6	4	3	U
OHURGENT	NEOM10DR10	NEO/POLY/HC OTIC 10ML SUS	6	4	4	U
OHURGENT	NITR100C47	NITROFURANTOIN BID 100MG CAP	6	10	8	U
OHURGENT	NITR0.4T35	NITROGLYCERIN 0.4MG/1TAB 25TAB BTL	6	50	32	U
OHURGENT	NITR1OIN2	NITROGLYCERIN 2% 1G OINT	6	0	4	U
OHURGENT	NYST10008	NYSTATIN ORAL 6000MU/60ML 60ML SUSP	6	0	1	U
OHURGENT	NYST100036	NYSTATIN SUSP 100000UNIT/1ML 5ML UDC	6	10	8	U
OHURGENT	OFLO5DRO9	OFLOXACIN 0.3% OPHTH 5ML SOL	6	5	3	U
OHURGENT	OMEP20CA60	OMEPRAZOLE 20MG CAP	6	10	6	U
OHURGENT	ONDA4DIS	ONDANSETRON 4MG/2ML 2ML INJ	6	10	9	U
OHURGENT	ONDA4TAB2	ONDANSETRON ODT 4MG TAB	6	20	20	U
OHURGENT	OSEL75CA	OSELTAMIVIR 75MG CAP	6	17	37	U
OHURGENT	OXYC1TAB13	oxyCODONE/ACETAMIN 5/325MG 1TAB TAB	2	20	18	U
OHURGENT	OXYM30SP86	OXYMETAZOLINE 0.05% NASAL 15ML BOTL	6	4	3	U
OHURGENT	PANT40VI2	PANTOPRAZOLE 40MG INJ	6	4	4	U
OHURGENT	PANT40TA3	PANTOPRAZOLE 40MG TAB	6	10	7	U
OHURGENT	PENI250T33	PENICILLIN VK 250MG TAB	6	10	10	U
OHURGENT	3710PEPKIT	PEP KIT 1 EACH	6	4	21	U
OHURGENT	PERM60CR	PERMETHRIN 5% CREAM 60G CRE	6	2	2	U
OHURGENT	PETR30JE	PETROLATUM 30G OINT	6	5	5	U
OHURGENT	PHEN-323	PHENAZOPYRIDINE 100MG TAB	6	10	7	U
OHURGENT	PHEN65VI2	PHENobarbital 65MG/1ML 1ML INJ	4	3	3	S

Appendix B

Limits: Omni Site+ID equals OHURGENT

Omni Site+ID	Item ID #	Item Description	Control Level	Par Level Qty	Qty On Hand	Stock Type
OHURGENT	POTA10CA2	POTASSIUM CHLORIDE 10MEQ TAB	6	10	9	U
OHURGENT	POVI473S	POVIDONE IODINE SOL 473ML SOL	6	10	10	U
OHURGENT	PRED15SO22	prednisoLONE 15MG/5ML 10ML SYP	6	50	50	U
OHURGENT	PRED5DRO18	prednisoLONE ACET 1% OPHTH 5ML SUS	6	4	4	U
OHURGENT	PRED10TA	predniSONE 10MG TAB	6	10	6	U
OHURGENT	PRED20TA	predniSONE 20MG TAB	6	10	8	U
OHURGENT	PRED5TAB3	predniSONE 5MG TAB	6	10	10	U
OHURGENT	PRED5SOL14	PRELONE 5MG/5ML 10ML SYP	6	40	40	U
OHURGENT	PROC25SU4	PROCHLORPERAZINE 25MG SUPP	6	10	9	U
OHURGENT	PROC5VIA11	PROCHLORPERAZINE 5MG/1ML 2ML ML	6	0	3	U
OHURGENT	PROM25SU8	PROMETHAZINE 25MG SUPP	6	5	3	U
OHURGENT	PROM25VI2	PROMETHAZINE 25MG/1ML 1ML INJ	6	10	6	U
OHURGENT	PSEU30TA36	PSEUDOEPHEDRINE 30MG TAB	6	10	11	U
OHURGENT	RABI150V2	RABIES IMMUNE GLOBULIN 10ML INJ	6	4	4	U
OHURGENT	RABI150V	RABIES IMMUNE GLOBULIN 2ML INJ	6	2	2	U
OHURGENT	RABI2.5K2	RABIES VACCINE 2.5U/1ML 1ML INJ	6	10	8	U
OHURGENT	RACE1VIA2	RACEPINEPHRINE 2.25% 0.5ML INH	0	5	5	U
OHURGENT	RANI-43	RANITIDINE 150MG TAB	6	10	10	U
OHURGENT	RANI50PI	RANITIDINE 50MG/50ML 50ML BAG	6	4	4	U
OHURGENT	3710FRIDGE	REFRIGERATOR ITEM 1EA/1EA 1EA INJ	6	999	999	U
OHURGENT	3710FREE2	RX BLANKS - PADS EACH	6	4	9	U
OHURGENT	3710FREE	RX BLANKS - ROLL EACH	6	2	3	U
OHURGENT	SODI45SP	SALINE NASAL 45ML SPRAY	6	2	2	U
OHURGENT	SULF1TAB32	SEPTRA DS 800/160MG 1EA TAB	6	10	6	U
OHURGENT	SILV1STI2	SILVER NITRATE APPLICATOR 1EA STICK	6	1	1	U
OHURGENT	SIME80TA10	SIMETHICONE 80MG CHEWABL	6	10	10	U
OHURGENT	SULF20OR	SMZ/TMP 800MG/160MG 20ML UDC	6	6	5	U
OHURGENT	SODI1DIS5	SOD BICARB 8.4% ABBOJECT 50ML INJ	6	0	4	S
OHURGENT	SODI1VIA3	SOD BICARB 8.4% VIAL 50ML INJ	6	2	2	U
OHURGENT	1/2100014	SOD CHLORIDE 0.45% 1000ML INJ	6	4	3	U
OHURGENT	NORM10006	SOD CHLORIDE 0.9% 1000ML INJ	6	12	11	U
OHURGENT	NORM100I10	SOD CHLORIDE 0.9% 100ML INJ	6	12	11	U
OHURGENT	NORM10VI2	SOD CHLORIDE 0.9% 10ML INJ	6	10	10	U
OHURGENT	NORM250I7	SOD CHLORIDE 0.9% 250ML INJ	6	4	4	U
OHURGENT	SODI3VIA4	SOD CHLORIDE 0.9% 3ML NEB	0	10	10	U
OHURGENT	NORM50IV8	SOD CHLORIDE 0.9% 50ML INJ	6	12	12	U
OHURGENT	NORM100P2	SOD CHLORIDE 0.9% ADD-VAN 100ML INJ	6	10	10	U
OHURGENT	NSADV50	SOD CHLORIDE 0.9% ADD-VAN 50ML INJ	6	10	10	U
OHURGENT	SODI15004	SOD CHLORIDE 0.9% IRRIG 1500ML SOL	6	0	12	U
OHURGENT	NSIRR500	SOD CHLORIDE 0.9% IRRIG 500ML SOL	6	24	23	U
OHURGENT	SULF15DR7	SOD SULFACETAMIDE 10% OPHTH 15ML SOL	6	4	3	U
OHURGENT	SILV50CR9	SSD CREAM 1% 50G CREAM	6	4	4	U
OHURGENT	WATE10VI	STERILE WATER 10ML INJ	6	10	9	U
OHURGENT	WATE500I5	STERILE WATER IRRIG 500ML BOTL	6	2	2	U
OHURGENT	SUMA6VIA4	SUMAtriptan 6MG/0.5ML 0.5ML INJ	6	5	3	U
OHURGENT	37103929	SURGILUBE PACKET 3G GEL	6	0	80	U

Limits: Omni Site+ID equals OHURGENT

Omni Site+ID	Item ID #	Item Description	Control Level	Par Level Qty	Qty On Hand	Stock Type
OHURGENT	DIPH0.5V9	TET ,DIPHTH,aPERT BOOSTRIX 0.5ML INJ	6	10	9	U
OHURGENT	TETA0.5D2	TET/DIPTHERIA ADULT VACC 0.5ML INJ	6	10	6	U
OHURGENT	TETA250D	TETANUS IMMUNE G 250UNITS/1ML 1ML INJ	6	2	2	U
OHURGENT	TETA5VIA2	TETANUS TOXOID VACCINE 0.5ML INJ	6	10	10	U
OHURGENT	TETR15DR22	TETRACAINE 0.5% OPHTH 15ML SOL	6	4	4	U
OHURGENT	BENZ0.66TI	TINCTURE BENZOIN 0.6ML UD 1EA TIN	6	10	9	U
OHURGENT	TOBR3.5O	TOBRAMYCIN 0.3% EYE 3.5G OINT	6	3	3	U
OHURGENT	TOBR5DRO12	TOBRAMYCIN 0.3% OPHTH 5ML SOL	6	4	4	U
OHURGENT	TRAM-34	traMADol 50MG TAB	6	10	10	U
OHURGENT	TRAM1TAB4	traMADol/ACETAMIN 37.5/325MG 1EA TAB	6	10	10	U
OHURGENT	VALA500T	valACYclovir 500MG TAB	6	10	6	U

END OF REPORT

Minimum Medication List

Oral

Ibuprofen 600 mg, pediatric suspension

Acetaminophen 325 mg, infant formula, pediatric suspension

Promethazine 25 mg PO, suppository

Acetaminophen-hydrocodone 500 mg/5 mg

Acetaminophen-oxycodone 325 mg/5 mg

Aspirin 81 mg

Amoxicillin 500 mg, 125 mg/5 cc, 250 mg/5 cc

Lorazepam

Diphenhydramine 25 mg, pediatric suspension

Ondansetron ODT, oral, intravenous

Cephalexin 500 mg

Clindamycin

Sulfamethoxazole-trimethoprim

Levofloxacin

Ciprofloxacin

Doxycycline

Azithromycin

Injectable

Ceftriaxone 1 gram

Clindamycin 600 mg

Epinephrine

Keratol ac 30/60 mg

Methylprednisolone

Morphine

Sodium chloride

Tetanus (Td/Tdap)

Other

Albuterol nebulizer solution

Albuterol inhaler

Example Patient Charge Master

5/17/11

EVALUATION AND MANAGEMENT

OFFICE VISIT	NEW	FEE	EST	FEE
NURSING CARE ONLY			99211	
PT LEVEL 1	99201		99211	
PT LEVEL 2	99202		99212	
PT LEVEL 3	99203		99213	
PT LEVEL 4	99204		99214	
PT LEVEL 5	99205		99215	

SELF PAY DISCOUNT - Quick Reference

NEW PT LEVEL 2	99202
NEW PT LEVEL 3	99203
NEW PT LEVEL 4	99204
NEW PT LEVEL 5	99205
EST PT LEVEL 2	99212
EST PT LEVEL 3	99213
EST PT LEVEL 4	99214
EST PT LEVEL 5	99215

Lee County School Emp. Physical: Do Not Bill Ins

TB TEST OR CHEST XRAY	N/A
PHYSICAL	N/A

Estero Mustang Football Physical: Do Not Bill Ins

PHYSICAL	N/A
EMERGENCY TRANSPORT	99058
SCHOOL PHYSICAL AGE 0-4	99382
SCHOOL PHYSICAL AGE 5-11	99383
WORK/SCHOOL PHYSICAL AGE 12-17	99384
WORK/SCHOOL PHYSICAL AGE 18-39	99385
PREVENTIVE COUNSELING - 15 MIN	99401
PREVENTIVE COUNSELING - 30 MIN	99402
DOT PHYSICAL	99455
TITMUS (VISUAL FIELD EXAM)	92081
PURE TONE AUDIOMETRY	92552

PROCEDURES

		FEE
ANTERIOR NOSEPACK	30901	
FOLEY URINARY CATHETER INSERTION	51702	
CATHETER SUPPLIES	A4314	
DENTAL BLOCK	64402	
MORGAN LENS	A4649	
DIGITAL BLOCK-CAN'T BILL IF BILLING FOR PROCEDURE	64450	

DEBRIDE - REMOVE

BURN 1ST DEGREE - SKIN CARE-INITIAL VISIT ONLY	16000
BURN 2ND / 3RD DEGREE DRESSING CHANGE OR DEBRIDEMENT (NO GLOBAL-CHARGE EACH VISIT)	16020
DEBRIDE SKIN, PARTIAL	11040
DEBRIDE SKIN, FULL THICKNESS	11041
DEBRIDE SKIN AND SUB-Q TISSUE	11042
DESTRUCT BENIGN LESION, 1-14 / WART	17110
FB REMOVAL (COMPLETE) - NOT FOOT - W/BLADE	10120
FB REMOVAL CONJUNCTIVA	65205
FB REMOVAL CORNEA W / 0 SLIT	65220
FB REMOVAL CORNEA W SLIT	65222
NAIL PLATE REMOVAL	11730
FB REMOVAL EXT AUDITORY CANAL (EAR)	69200
FB REMOVAL INTRANASAL (NOSE)	30300
CERUMEN REMOVAL W/ INSTRUMENT	69210

INCISE - DRAIN - ASPIRATE

I & D ABSCESS SKIN - SIMPLE	10060
I & D ABSCESS SKIN - (Complex or >1)	10061
I & D HEMATOMA / SEROMA / FLUID	10140
I & D EYELID - BLEPHAR	67700
I & D PARONYCCHIA / FINGER ABSCESS	26010
I & D PERIANAL ABSCESS	46050
I & D PILONIDAL CYST	10080
INCISE EXTERNAL HEMORRHOID	46083
ASPIRATE ABSCESS, HEMATOMA, BULLA CYST	10160
ASPIRATE BURSA ELBOW (OR INTERMEDIATE JOINT)	20605
ASPIRATE KNEE (OR MAJOR BURSA)	20610
SUBUNGUAL HEMATOMA EVACUATION	11740

RESP / CARDIAC

PULSE OX	94760
NEB TREATMENT	94640
NEB SUPPLIES	A7003
SPIROMETRY	94010
SPIROMETRY PRE+POST NEB TX	94060
CHEST WALL PERCUSSION - CUPPING, INITIAL	94667
CHEST WALL PERCUSSION, SUBSEQ., SAME VISIT	94668
MDI DEMO / EVAL PT USAGE	94664
EKG	93000

LABORATORY

SPECIMEN HANDLING / SEND OUT UDS - SEND OUT ONLY	99000
UDS - SEND WITH OUR COC FORM	80100
UDS - RAPID	80100R
ALCOHOL BREATH (BAT)	82075
ACCUCHECK	82962QW
BASIC METABOLIC PANEL	80048QW
CMP	80053QW
H. PYLORI	83009QW
HEMOGLOBIN	85018QW
INR / PT	85610QW
INFLUENZA A&B (Bill for both seperately)	87804QW
MONOSPOT	86308QW
RAPID STREP	87880QW
URINE DIP	81002QW
URINE PREG.	81025QW
TB / PPD	86580

IMMUNIZATION & VACCINATIONS

IMMUNIZATION INJECTION FEE	90471
TD VACCINE	90718
INFLUENZA VACCINE INJ. FEE	G0008
INFLUENZA VACCINE	90658
HEPATITIS A INJECTION FEE	90471
HEPATITIS A VACCINE	90632
HEPATITIS B INJECTION FEE	G0010
HEPATITIS B VACCINE	90746
PNEUMOCOCCAL INJECTION FEE	G0009

The Healthcare Executive's Guide to Urgent Care Centers and Freestanding EDs

X-RAY

	Code
ABDOMEN / KUB	74000
ACUTE ABDOMINAL SERIES	74022
ANKLE	73610
C SPINE, 3 VIEWS	72040
C SPINE, 5 VIEWS	72050
CALCANEOUS, 2 VIEWS	73650
CHEST, PA & LAT	71020
ELBOW	73080
FINGER(S)	73140
FOOT	73630
FOREARM, AP & LAT	73090
HAND, 3 VIEWS	73130
HIP	73510
HIPS (BILATERAL)	73520
HUMERUS, 2 VIEWS	73060
KNEE, PA & LAT	73560
KNEE W/ PATELLA (>3 VIEW)	73562
L SPINE, 2-3 VIEWS	72100
L SPINE, 4-5 VIEWS	72110
NASAL BONES	70160
NECK / SOFT TISSUE	70360
PELVIS	72170
RIBS	71101
SACRUM / COCCYX	72220
SHOULDER	73030
TIB-FIB	73590
TOE(S)	73660
T SPINE (2 VIEWS)	72070
WRIST (3 VIEW)	73110

Additional Charges:

ORTHO ***FILL OUT BORON SHEET***

	Code
CRUTCHES / GAIT TRAINING	97116
FINGER SPLINT (Stacked/Protector)	A4570
FINGER SPLINT (CUSTOM)	29130
SHORTARM SPLINT (CUSTOM)	29125
LONG ARM SPLINT (CUSTOM)	29105
LOWER LEG SPLINT (CUSTOM)	29515
RADIAL HEAD SUBLUXATION	24640
MODERATE SEDATION	99144
SHOULDER DISLOCATION	23650
OSTEOPATHIC MANIPULATION	98925

Simple Closure - Scalp, Axillae, Trunk, Extremities

	Code
DERMABOND (MEDICARE PATIENT ONLY)	G0168
< = 2.5 cm	12001
2.6 - 7.5 cm	12002
7.6 to 12.5	12004

Layered Closure - Scalp, Axillae, Trunk, Extremities

	Code
< = 2.5 cm	12031
2.6 - 7.5 cm	12032
7.6 - 12.5 cm	12034

Layered Closure of Wounds of Neck, Hands, Feet

	Code
< = 2.5 cm	12041
2.6 - 7.5 cm	12042
7.6 - 12.5 cm	12044

Simple Closure of Face, Ears, Eyelids, Nose, Lips

	Code
< = 2.5 cm	12011
2.6 - 5.0 cm	12013
5.1 - 7.5 cm	12014

Layered Closure of Face, Ears, Eyelids, Nose, Lips

	Code
< = 2.5 cm	12051
2.6 - 5.0 cm	12052
5.1 - 7.5 cm	12053

INFUSION / INJECTIONS

	Code	#	Per Unit	Total
INJECTION IM / SUBQ (1 PER DOSE)	96372			
HEP LOCK - NO MEDS OR FLUIDS	A4221			
IV PUSH INITIAL	96374			
IV PUSH EACH ADD'L DOSE OF DIFF MED	96375			
IV PUSH EACH ADD'L DOSE OF SAME MED	96376			
HYDRATION IV 1ST HOUR	96360			
HYDRATION IV EACH ADD. HOUR	96361			
MED. IV INFUSION, INITIAL	96365			
MED. IV INFUSION, EACH NEW MED	96366			

MEDICATION / FLUID

	Code	#	Per Unit	Total
ALBUTEROL UP TO 2.5 MG	J7620			
ATROVENT UP TO 1MG	J7644			
ANCEF INJECTION PER 500MG	J0690			
ATIVAN	J2060			
BENADRYL 50 MG	J1200			
DECADRON PER 1MG	J1100			
DEMEROL PER 100MG	J2175			
DILAUDID UP TO 4MG	J1170			
EPINEPHRINE UP TO 1ML	J0170			
FENTANYL PER 0.1MG	J3010			
MORPHINE UP TO 10MG	J2270			
NORFLEX 60 MG, IV, IM	J2360			
PEPCID 20MG, IV	S0028			
PHENERGAN (50 MG)	J2550			
REGLAN INJ UP TO 10MG	J2765			
ROCEPHIN INJ 250MG	J0696			
ROCEPHIN INJ 500MG	J0696			
ROCEPHIN INJ 1GM	J0696			
SOLUMEDROL UP TO 125MG	J2930			
TORADOL PER 30MG	J1885			
VERSED PER 1MG	J2250			
VITAMIN B-12	J3420			
NS 1000 ml 1000ml	J7030			
D5.45 1000ml	J7042			